T0269244

Clinicians' Guides to Radionuclide Hybrid Imaging

Series editors:
Jamshed B. Bomanji
London, UK

Gopinath Gnanasegaran
London, UK

Stefano Fanti
Bologna, Italy

Homer A. Macapinlac
Houston, Texas, USA

More information about this series at http://www.springer.com/series/13803

Tara Barwick • Andrea Rockall
Editors

PET/CT in Gynecological Cancers

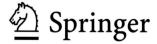 Springer

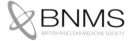

Editors
Tara Barwick
Imperial College Healthcare NHS Trust
London, UK

Department of Surgery and Cancer
Imperial College
London, UK

Andrea Rockall
Imperial College Healthcare NHS Trust
London, UK

Department of Surgery and Cancer
Imperial College
London, UK

ISSN 2367-2439   ISSN 2367-2447   (electronic)
Clinicians' Guides to Radionuclide Hybrid Imaging - PET/CT
ISBN 978-3-319-29247-2   ISBN 978-3-319-29249-6   (eBook)
DOI 10.1007/978-3-319-29249-6

Library of Congress Control Number: 2016940198

© Springer International Publishing Switzerland 2016
This work is subject to copyright. All rights are reserved by the Publisher, whether the whole or part of the material is concerned, specifically the rights of translation, reprinting, reuse of illustrations, recitation, broadcasting, reproduction on microfilms or in any other physical way, and transmission or information storage and retrieval, electronic adaptation, computer software, or by similar or dissimilar methodology now known or hereafter developed.
The use of general descriptive names, registered names, trademarks, service marks, etc. in this publication does not imply, even in the absence of a specific statement, that such names are exempt from the relevant protective laws and regulations and therefore free for general use.
The publisher, the authors and the editors are safe to assume that the advice and information in this book are believed to be true and accurate at the date of publication. Neither the publisher nor the authors or the editors give a warranty, express or implied, with respect to the material contained herein or for any errors or omissions that may have been made.

Printed on acid-free paper

This Springer imprint is published by Springer Nature
The registered company is Springer International Publishing AG Switzerland

Foreword

Clear and concise clinical indications for PET/CT in the management of the oncology patient are presented in this series of 15 separate Booklets.

The impact on better staging, tailored management and specific treatment of the patient with cancer has been achieved with the advent of this multimodality imaging technology. Early and accurate diagnosis will always pay, and clear information can be gathered with PET/CT on treatment responses. Prognostic information is gathered and can forward guide additional therapeutic options.

It is a fortunate coincidence that PET/CT was able to derive great benefit from radionuclide-labelled probes, which deliver good and often excellent target to non-target signals. Whilst labelled glucose remains the cornerstone for the clinical benefit achieved, a number of recent probes are definitely adding benefit. PET/CT is hence an evolving technology, extending its applications and indications. Significant advances in the instrumentation and data processing available have also contributed to this technology, which delivers high throughput and a wealth of data, with good patient tolerance and indeed patient and public acceptance. As an example, the role of PET/CT in the evaluation of cardiac disease is also covered, with emphasis on labelled rubidium and labelled glucose studies.

The novel probes of labelled choline, labelled peptides, such as DOTATATE, and, most recently, labelled PSMA (prostate-specific membrane antigen) have gained rapid clinical utility and acceptance, as significant PET/CT tools for the management of neuroendocrine disease and prostate cancer patients, notwithstanding all the advances achieved with other imaging modalities, such as MRI. Hence a chapter reviewing novel PET tracers forms part of this series.

The oncological community has recognised the value of PET/CT and has delivered advanced diagnostic criteria for some of the most important indications for PET/CT. This includes the recent Deauville criteria for the classification of PET/CT patients with lymphoma – similar criteria are expected to develop for other malignancies, such as head and neck cancer, melanoma and pelvic malignancies. For completion, a separate section covers the role of PET/CT in radiotherapy planning, discussing the indications for planning biological tumour volumes in relevant cancers.

These Booklets offer simple, rapid and concise guidelines on the utility of PET/CT in a range of oncological indications. They also deliver a rapid aide memoire on the merits and appropriate indications for PET/CT in oncology.

London, UK   Peter J. Ell, FMedSci, DR HC, AΩA

Preface

Hybrid Imaging with PET/CT and SPECT/CT combines best of function and structure to provide accurate localisation, characterisation and diagnosis. There is extensive literature and evidence to support PET/CT, which has made significant impact in oncological imaging and management of patients with cancer. The evidence in favour of SPECT/CT especially in orthopaedic indications is evolving and increasing.

The Clinicians' Guides to Radionuclide Hybrid Imaging pocketbook series is specifically aimed at our referring clinicians, nuclear medicine/radiology doctors, radiographers/technologists, and nurses who are routinely working in nuclear medicine and participate in Multi-Disciplinary Meetings. This series is the joint work of many friends and professionals from different nations who share a common dream and vision towards promoting and supporting nuclear medicine as a useful and important imaging speciality.

We want to thank all those people who have contributed to this work as advisors, authors and reviewers, without whom the book would not have been possible. We want to thank our members from the BNMS (British Nuclear Medicine Society, UK) for their encouragement and support, and we are extremely grateful to Dr Brian Nielly, Charlotte Weston, the BNMS Education Committee and the BNMS council members for their enthusiasm and trust.

Finally, we wish to extend particular gratitude to the industry for their continuous supports towards education and training.

London, UK   Gopinath Gnanasegaran
                                                                           Jamshed Bomanji

Acknowledgements

The series co-ordinators and editors would like to express sincere gratitude to the members of the British Nuclear Medicine Society, patients, teachers, colleagues, students, the industry and the BNMS Education Committee Members, for their continued support and inspiration:

Andy Bradley
Brent Drake
Francis Sundram
James Ballinger
Parthiban Arumugam
Rizwan Syed
Sai Han
Vineet Prakash

Contents

Contributors

Kanhaiyalal Agrawal Department of Nuclear Medicine and PET/CT, North City Hospital, Kolkata, India

James Ballinger Division of Imaging Sciences, King's College London, London, UK

Tara Barwick Imperial College Healthcare NHS Trust, London, UK

Department of Surgery and Cancer, Imperial College, London, UK

Nishat Bharwani Department of Surgery & Cancer, Imperial College London, UK

Department of Imaging, St Mary's Hospital, Imperial College Healthcare NHS Trust, London, UK

Jamshed Bomanji Department of Nuclear Medicine, University College London Hospitals NHS Foundation Trust, London, UK

Jane Borley Department of Gynaecology Oncology, Division Women and Children's Health, Hammersmith Hospital, Imperial College Healthcare NHS Trust, London, UK

Andy Bradley Nuclear Medicine Centre, Manchester Royal Infirmary, Manchester, UK

Alexis Corrigan Department of Nuclear Medicine and Radiology, Maidstone and Tunbridge Wells NHS Trust, Tunbridge Wells, UK

John Dickson Department of Nuclear Medicine, Nuclear Medicine Centre, University College London Hospitals NHS Foundation Trust, London, UK

Sadaf Ghaem-Maghami Department of Gynaecology Oncology, Division Women and Children's Health, Imperial College London, Imperial College Healthcare NHS Trust, London, UK

Gopinath Gnanasegaran Department of Nuclear Medicine, Royal Free London NHS Foundation Trust, London, UK

Sharanpal Jeetle Department of Cellular Pathology, Bart's Health NHS Trust, London, UK

Sairah R. Khan Department of Radiology, Imperial College Healthcare NHS Trust, Charing Cross Hospital, London, UK

Shaunak Navalkissoor Department of Nuclear Medicine, Royal Free London NHS Foundation Trust, London, UK

Nicholas Reed Department of Clinical Oncology, Beatson Oncology Centre, Gartnavel General Hospital, Glasgow, Scotland

Azmat Sadozye Department of Clinical Oncology, Beatson Oncology Centre, Gartnavel General Hospital, Glasgow, Scotland

Naveena Singh Department of Cellular Pathology, Bart's Health NHS Trust, London, UK

Evangelia Skoura Department of Nuclear Medicine, Institute of Nuclear Medicine, UCLH, London, UK

Victoria Stewart Department of Radiology, Imperial College Healthcare NHS Trust, Charing Cross Hospital, London, UK

Teresa A. Szyszko Division of Imaging Sciences and Biomedical Engineering, Nuclear Medicine and Radiology Clinical PET Centre, St Thomas' Hospital, Kings College London, London, UK

Deborah Tout Biomedical Technology Services, Gold Coast University Hospital, Southport, QLD, Australia

Thomas Wagner Department of Nuclear Medicine, Royal Free London NHS Foundation Trust, London, UK

Gynaecological Malignancies: Epidemiology, Clinical Presentation, Diagnosis, Staging and Staging Procedures

Jane Borley and Sadaf Ghaem-Maghami

Contents

J. Borley, PhD, MRCOG
Department of Gynaecology Oncology, Division Women and Children's Health,
Hammersmith Hospital, Imperial College Healthcare NHS Trust, London, UK
e-mail: j.borley10@imperial.ac.uk

S. Ghaem-Maghami, PhD, MRCOG (✉)
Department of Gynaecology Oncology, Division Women and Children's Health,
Imperial College London, Imperial College Healthcare NHS Trust, London, UK
e-mail: s.ghaem-maghami@imperial.ac.uk

© Springer International Publishing Switzerland 2016
T. Barwick, A. Rockall (eds.), *PET/CT in Gynecological Cancers*,
Clinicians' Guides to Radionuclide Hybrid Imaging, DOI 10.1007/978-3-319-29249-6_1

1.1 Cervical Cancer

1.1.1 Epidemiology

Cervical cancer is the 12th most common cancer in women in the UK with 3064 new cases in 2011 [3]; however, globally it is the 3rd most common cancer in women with 530,000 new cases reported in 2008 [6]. Age-specific incidence is highest in those aged 30–34 with a second peak in those aged 80–84. The overall 5-year survival rate is 67% [3].

1.1.2 Classification

The majority of cervical tumours are squamous cell (80%) originating from the squamous epithelium or adenocarcinomas (10–15%) from the glandular epithelium, both subtypes are treated identically. Other rarer forms of cervical cancer include clear cell and small cell carcinomas.

1.1.3 Aetiology

Persistent human papillomavirus (HPV) infection is attributable to almost all cases of cervical cancer, with high-risk subtypes 16 and 18 being the most prevalent [1]. HPV invades cervical epithelium and produces viral oncoproteins which interfere with cell cycle regulation genes such as p53 and Rb. [10]. Smoking and immuno-suppression increase the risk of cervical cancer as a result of less effective HPV clearance. Vaccination to both high- and low-risk HPV is effective when given pre-exposure.

The natural pathology of HPV to cervical cancer has been clearly documented; persistent HPV infection leads to cervical intraepithelial neoplasia which in turn can progress to early invasive cancer (microinvasion) and subsequently metastatic cervical cancer. The NHS cervical screening programme is designed to detect these preinvasive changes which is estimated to have saved 100,000 lives since its introduction in 1988 [12].

1.1.4 Clinical Presentation

Presentation may be asymptomatic with disease identified through the national cervical cytology screening programme, following treatment for high-grade intraepithelial neoplasia (CIN2-3), or incidentally during gynaecological examination with classic examination findings of a hard, craggy, bleeding cervix. Symptoms of cervical cancer are related to the tumour itself and may present as symptoms of vaginal bleeding, menorrhagia, intermenstrual or post-coital bleeding or may present with advanced progression such as renal failure following ureteric obstruction.

Table 1.1 FIGO staging of cervical cancer

Stage 1	*Tumour confined to the cervix*
1A	Invasive carcinoma only diagnosed on microscopy
1A1	Stromal invasion ≤3 mm in depth and ≤7 mm in length
1A2	Stromal invasion >3 mm but ≤5 mm in depth and ≤7 mm in length
1B	Clinically visible tumours or microinvasive tumours that are >5 mm in depth and/or >7 mm in length
1B1	Tumour ≤4 cm in greatest dimension
1B2	Tumour >4 cm in greatest dimension
Stage 2	*Tumour invades beyond the uterus but not to the pelvic sidewall or lower third of the vagina*
Stage 2A	Tumour does not invade to the parametrium
2A1	Tumour ≤4 cm in greatest dimension
2A2	Tumour >4 cm in greatest dimension
Stage 2B	Tumour has spread to the parametrium
Stage 3	*Tumour extends to the pelvic wall and/or the lower third of the vagina*
3A	Tumour extends to the lower third of the vagina without pelvic wall involvement
3B	Extension to the pelvic wall and/or hydronephrosis or non-functioning kidney
Stage 4	*Tumour has spread beyond the true pelvis and/or biopsy-proven extension to the bladder or rectum*
4A	Spread to adjacent organs
4B	Spread to distant organs

1.1.5   Diagnosis

Clinically suspected tumours require cervical biopsy for histopathological diagnosis. Examination under anaesthesia with cystoscopy, +/−hysteroscopy or sigmoidoscopy aims to stage the tumour. Imaging (pelvic MRI, chest CT, abdominal and pelvic +/−FDG PET/CT) is used to assess spread to other organs as detailed in Chaps. 4 and 9.

1.1.6   Staging

Staging is defined by FIGO (Federation of Gynecology and Obstetrics) [11]. See Table 1.1.

1.2   Endometrial Cancer

1.2.1   Epidemiology

Endometrial cancer is the most common gynaecological malignancy and the 4th most common female cancer in the UK. In 2011 there were 8475 new cases in the UK [4]. The incidence has increased by 48 % in the past 15 years, attributable to the increase in obesity and changes to reproductive practices [5]. The 5-year overall survival rate is 77.3 % [4].

1.2.2 Classification

Eighty to eighty-five percent of endometrial carcinomas are endometrioid adeno-carcinomas, 10 % are papillary serous and 4 % are clear cell.

1.2.3 Aetiology

The majority of risk factors for endometrial cancer are associated with excessive oestrogens which can be endogenous such as in obesity, early menarche and late menopause, nulliparity and oestrogen-secreting tumours or exogenous oestrogens such as in tamoxifen therapy and hormone replacement therapy (HRT). Age, endometrial hyperplasia and genetic factors such as Lynch syndrome also increase risk.

1.2.4 Clinical Presentation

The majority of women (>90 %) present with episodes of postmenopausal bleeding but may also present with persistent vaginal discharge, symptoms of metastases or incidentally through other investigations. Cervical smear tests which report endometrial cells or glandular abnormalities may warrant investigation of endometrial cancer.

1.2.5 Diagnosis

Those presenting with postmenopausal bleeding should undergo transvaginal ultrasound scan to visualise the endometrial cavity. Those without HRT and an endometrial thickness of >3 mm or (>5 mm in those taking sequential HRT) should have endometrial sampling through endometrial pipelle biopsy or hysteroscopy and curettage [15]. Following a diagnosis of endometrial cancer, staging investigations include MRI of the pelvis and CT of the chest, abdomen and pelvis (Chap. 4).

1.2.6 Staging

Staging is defined by FIGO (Federation of Gynecology and Obstetrics) [11]. See Table 1.2.

Table 1.2 FIGO staging of endometrial cancer

Stage 1	*Tumour confined to the corpus uteri or endocervical glandular involvement*
1A	<50 % invasion of the myometrium
1B	≥50 % invasion of the myometrium
Stage 2	*Tumour invades the cervical stroma but does not extend beyond the uterus*
Stage 3	*Local and/or regional spread of tumour*
3A	Tumour invades the serosa of the corpus uteri and/or adnexa
3B	Vagina and/or parametrial involvement
3C	Metastasis to pelvic and/or para-aortic lymph nodes
	(i) Positive pelvic lymph nodes
	(ii) Positive para-aortic lymph nodes with or without positive pelvic lymph nodes
Stage 4	*Tumour invades the bladder and/or bowel mucosa and/or distant metastases*
4A	Tumour invades the bladder and/or bowel mucosa
4B	Distant metastases, including intra-abdominal metastases and/or inguinal lymph nodes

1.3   Ovarian Cancer

1.3.1   Epidemiology

Ovarian cancer is the second most common gynaecological malignancy and the fifth most common cause of cancer in women. In 2010 over 7000 women were diagnosed with the disease in the UK, and it caused 4295 deaths in the same year [2]. The incidence of ovarian cancer increases after the menopause with the peak incidence in those aged 60–64 years of age. Unlike other gynaecological cancers, due to the late presentation of the disease, overall survival is very poor with only 34 % of patients surviving 5 years after their diagnosis [14].

1.3.2   Classification

Ovarian cancer is broadly classified into three distinct histological categories: epithelial, germ cell (dysgerminoma, immature teratoma and yolk sac tumours) and sex cord-stromal tumours (granulosa cell tumour, Sertoli-Leydig cell tumours). The majority (90 %) of ovarian cancers are epithelial in origin. They can be further categorised in their subtypes: high-grade serous (most common), endometrioid, clear cell, mucinous and low-grade serous [7].

1.3.3 Aetiology

Increasing age and known genetic mutations are thought to be the most important risk factors for developing OC [2]. Women with BRCA1 and BRCA2 mutations have a risk of developing OC by the age of 70 of between 40–59 % and 16.5–18 %, respectively [9]. Women with hereditary nonpolyposis colorectal cancer (HNPCC) have a 6.7 % lifetime risk of developing OC [16]. However, only 10 % of patients with OC have a family history of the disease and in those known genetic mutations account for less than 50 %. Reproductive factors are also known to affect the risk of developing OC with an increased risk found in those with early menarche and late menopause and nulliparity. Conversely pregnancy, breastfeeding and the combined oral contraceptive pill are found to be protective.

1.3.4 Clinical Presentation

The majority of cases present with advanced disease with symptoms being insidious and nonspecific such as abdominal or pelvic pain, abdominal bloating, difficulty in eating or early satiety, increased urinary urgency/frequency, unexplained weight loss, fatigue or changes in bowel habit. Others may present with an incidental finding of a suspicious cyst on ultrasound scan. Sex cord-stromal tumours may secrete unopposed oestrogens and therefore may present as precious puberty, postmenopausal bleeding or menorrhagia.

1.3.5 Diagnosis

Diagnosis is based on histopathology, but often a high risk of malignancy is suspected based on the appearances of the cyst on ultrasound [8], CA 125 blood levels and presence of metastasis on further imaging or at the time of surgery.

1.3.6 Staging

Staging is defined by FIGO (Federation of Gynecology and Obstetrics) [13]. See Table 1.3.

Table 1.3 FIGO staging of ovarian tumours

Stage 1	*Tumour confined to the ovaries or fallopian tube(s)*
1A	Tumour limited to one ovary (capsule intact) or fallopian tube, no malignant cells in ascites or peritoneal washings, no tumour on ovarian or fallopian tube surface
1B	Tumour limited to both ovaries (capsule intact) or fallopian tubes, no malignant cells in ascites or peritoneal washings, no tumour on ovarian or fallopian tube surface
1C	Tumour limited to one or both ovaries or fallopian tubes with either Surgical spill of cyst contents Capsule ruptured before surgery or tumour on the ovary/fallopian tube surface Malignant cells in ascites or peritoneal washings
Stage 2	*Tumour involves one or both ovaries or fallopian tubes with pelvic extension (below the pelvic brim) or primary peritoneal cancer*
2A	Extension and/or implants on the uterus and/or fallopian tubes and/or ovaries
2B	Extension to other pelvic intraperitoneal tissues
Stage 3	*Tumour involves one or both ovaries or fallopian tubes or primary peritoneal cancer, with cytologically or histologically confirmed spread to the peritoneum outside the pelvis and/or metastasis to retroperitoneal lymph nodes*
3A1	Positive retroperitoneal lymph nodes only (i) Metastasis ≤10 mm in greatest dimension (ii) Metastasis >10 mm in greatest dimension
3A2	Microscopic extrapelvic peritoneal involvement with or without positive retroperitoneal lymph nodes
3B	Macroscopic peritoneal metastasis beyond the pelvis ≤2 cm in greatest diameter, with or without positive retroperitoneal lymph nodes
3C	Macroscopic peritoneal metastasis beyond the pelvis >2 cm in greatest diameter, with or without positive retroperitoneal lymph nodes. Includes extension of tumour to capsule of the liver and spleen without parenchymal involvement
Stage 4	*Distant metastasis excluding peritoneal metastasis*
4A	Pleural effusion with positive cytology
4B	Parenchymal metastases and metastases to extra-abdominal organs (including inguinal lymph nodes and lymph nodes outside the abdominal cavity)

Key Points

Cervical Cancer

The majority of cervical tumours are squamous cell.

Persistent human papillomavirus (HPV) infection is attributable to almost all cases of cervical cancer.

Symptoms of cervical cancer are related to the tumour itself (vaginal bleeding, menorrhagia, intermenstrual or post-coital bleeding or renal failure following ureteric obstruction in advanced stage).

Clinically suspected tumours require cervical biopsy for histopathological diagnosis.

Endometrial Cancer

Majority of endometrial carcinomas are endometrioid adenocarcinomas (80–85 %).

Excessive endogenous oestrogen (eg. obesity) is the main risk factor for endometrial cancer.

Majority of women (>90 %) present with episodes of postmenopausal bleeding.

Patients with postmenopausal bleeding should undergo transvaginal ultrasound scan to determine endometrial thickness.

Ovarian Cancer

Ovarian cancer is the second most common gynaecological malignancy and the fifth most common cause of cancer in women.

Overall survival is very poor with only 34 % of patients surviving 5 years after their diagnosis.

Majority (90 %) of ovarian cancers are epithelial in origin.

Increasing age and known genetic mutations are thought to be the most important risk factors.

The majority of cases present with advanced disease with symptoms being insidious and nonspecific.

Diagnosis is based on histopathology.

References

1. Bosch FX, Lorincz A, Munoz N, Meijer CJ, Shah KV. The causal relation between human papillomavirus and cervical cancer. J Clin Pathol. 2002;55:244–65.
2. Cancer Research UK. Cancer statistics report: ovarian cancer. UK: Cancer Research UK; 2011.
3. Cancer Research UK. Cancer statistics report: cervical cancer. UK: Cancer Research UK; 2014.
4. Cancer Research UK. Cancer statistics report: uterine cancer. UK: Cancer Research UK; 2014.
5. Evans T, Sany O, Pearmain P, Ganesan R, Blann A, Sundar S. Differential trends in the rising incidence of endometrial cancer by type: data from a UK population-based registry from 1994 to 2006. Br J Cancer. 2011;104:1505–10.
6. Ferlay J, Shin HR, Bray F, Forman D, Mathers C, Parkin DM. Estimates of worldwide burden of cancer in 2008: GLOBOCAN 2008. Int J Cancer. 2010;127:2893–917.
7. Gurung A, Hung T, Morin J, Gilks CB. Molecular abnormalities in ovarian carcinoma: clinical, morphological and therapeutic correlates. Histopathology. 2013;62:59–70.
8. Kaijser J, Bourne T, Valentin L, Sayasneh A, Van Holsbeke C, Vergote I, Testa AC, Franchi D, Van Calster B, Timmerman D. Improving strategies for diagnosing ovarian cancer: a summary of the International Ovarian Tumor Analysis (IOTA) studies. Ultrasound Obstet Gynecol. 2013;41:9–20.
9. Mavaddat N, Peock S, Frost D, Ellis S, Platte R, Fineberg E, Evans DG, Izatt L, Eeles RA, Adlard J, Davidson R, Eccles D, Cole T, Cook J, Brewer C, Tischkowitz M, Douglas F, Hodgson S, Walker L, Porteous ME, Morrison PJ, Side LE, Kennedy MJ, Houghton C,

Donaldson A, Rogers MT, Dorkins H, Miedzybrodzka Z, Gregory H, Eason J, Barwell J, Mccann E, Murray A, Antoniou AC, Easton DF. Cancer risks for BRCA1 and BRCA2 mutation carriers: results from prospective analysis of EMBRACE. J Natl Cancer Inst. 2013;105:812–22.

10. Mighty KK, Laimins LA. The role of human papillomaviruses in oncogenesis. Recent Results Cancer Res. 2014;193:135–48.

11. Pecorelli S. Revised FIGO staging for carcinoma of the vulva, cervix, and endometrium. Int J Gynaecol Obstet. 2009;105:103–4.

12. Peto J, Gilham C, Fletcher O, Matthews FE. The cervical cancer epidemic that screening has prevented in the UK. Lancet. 2004;364:249–56.

13. Prat J, Oncology, F. C. O. G. Staging classification for cancer of the ovary, fallopian tube, and peritoneum. Int J Gynaecol Obstet. 2014;124:1–5.

14. Ries LAG, Young JL, Keel GE, Eisner MP, Lin YD, Horner M-J (editors). SEER Survival Monograph: Cancer Survival Among Adults: U.S. SEER Program, 1988–2001, Patient and Tumor Characteristics. National Cancer Institute, SEER Program, NIH Pub. No. 07-6215, Bethesda, MD, 2007.

15. Scottish Intercollegiate Guidelines Network. Investigation of postmenopausal bleeding. Edinburgh: SIGN Publication; 2002. p. 61.

16. Watson P, Vasen HF, Mecklin JP, Bernstein I, Aarnio M, Jarvinen HJ, Myrhoj T, Sunde L, Wijnen JT, Lynch HT. The risk of extra-colonic, extra-endometrial cancer in the Lynch syndrome. Int J Cancer. 2008;123:444–9.

An Overview of the Pathology of Gynaecological Cancers

2

Naveena Singh and Sharanpal Jeetle

Contents

2.1   Cervix

HPV-related cancers are preceded by intraepithelial neoplasias within cervical squamous or glandular epithelium in the transformation zone; these are invisible to the naked eye. Carcinomas of the cervix (Table 2.1) are exophytic (polypoidal/papillary), ulcerative or endophytic, commonly resulting in a hard, barrel-shaped cervix.

Squamous cell carcinoma (SCC) shows sheets or nests of polygonal, squamous cells invading the underlying cervical stroma. The squamous cells are characterised by glassy pink cytoplasm and intercellular bridges. Pearls of keratin or keratohyaline granules are evident in *keratinizing* SCC (Fig. 2.1). *Basaloid SCC* is composed of cells that have scanty cytoplasm and dark, irregular nuclei and show large geographic areas of tumour necrosis. *Verrucous SCC* is a low-grade tumour with a hyperkeratotic, undulating surface and minimal cytological atypia and a pushing rather than infiltrative invasive front. *Warty (condylomatous) SCC* looks similar but with more atypical cytological features of viral infection (koilocytosis).

N. Singh (✉) • S. Jeetle
Department of Cellular Pathology, Bart's Health NHS Trust, London, UK
e-mail: N.Singh@bartshealth.nhs.uk; s.jeetle@bartshealth.nhs.uk

© Springer International Publishing Switzerland 2016   11
T. Barwick, A. Rockall (eds.), *PET/CT in Gynecological Cancers*,
Clinicians' Guides to Radionuclide Hybrid Imaging, DOI 10.1007/978-3-319-29249-6_2

Table 2.1 WHO classification of malignant cervical tumours

WHO classification of malignant cervical tumours
Squamous cell carcinoma
Keratinising
Non-keratinising
Papillary
Basaloid
Warty
Verrucous
Squamotransitional
Lymphoepithelioma-like
Adenocarcinoma
Endocervical, usual type
Mucinous (gastric, intestinal, signet ring subtypes)
Villoglandular
Endometrioid
Clear Cell
Serous
Mesonephric
Mixed adenocarcinoma/neuroendocrine
Other epithelial malignancies
Adenosquamous
Adenoid basal
Adenoid cystic
Undifferentiated
Neuroendocrine
Low grade (carcinoid, atypical carcinoid)
High grade (large cell, small cell)
Mesenchymal
Leiomyosarcoma
Rhabdomyosarcoma
Alveolar soft part sarcoma
Angiosarcoma
Malignant peripheral nerve sheath tumour
Others (liposarcoma, undifferentiated endocervical carcinoma, Ewing sarcoma)
Malignant mixed tumours
Adenosarcoma
Carcinosarcoma
Others
Malignant melanoma
Yolk sac tumour
Lymphoma
Secondary deposits from other sites

Adenocarcinoma is a malignancy of glandular mucosa which is usually associated with HPV, although a minority (including those of gastric type) are HPV independent. *Endocervical adenocarcinoma, usual type*, is architecturally complex and composed of coalescing round to oval glands lined by endocervical-type cells possessing frequent mitotic figures and necrosis (Fig. 2.2). *Mucinous tumours* are composed of malignant cells which may demonstrate goblet cell

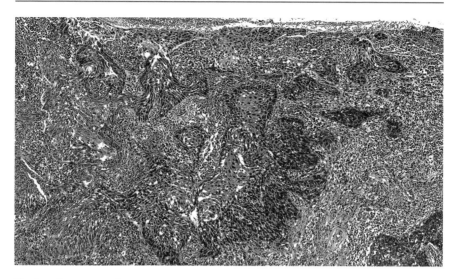

Fig. 2.1 Squamous cell carcinoma characterised by haphazard proliferation of islands of malignant squamous epithelium showing central keratinisation

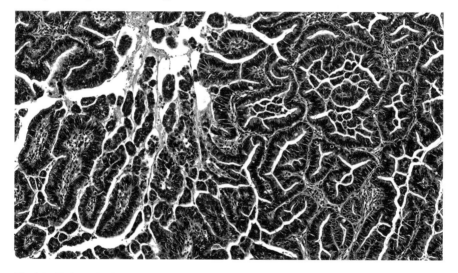

Fig. 2.2 Endocervical adenocarcinoma seen as a complex glandular proliferation of cells showing cytological atypia

morphology (*intestinal type*), signet ring morphology (*signet ring type*) or cells of stomach lining (*gastric type*, including *adenoma malignum*; the latter subtype is infiltrative but morphologically bland and may show prominent cystically dilated glands). *Villoglandular carcinoma* demonstrates a predominantly exophytic papillary growth pattern composed of endocervical-type cells. *Endometrioid carcinoma* is a rare subtype resembling typical endometrial carcinoma.

Adenosquamous carcinoma shows combined morphological features of SCC and adenocarcinoma.

Neuroendocrine tumours are currently classified as low-grade or high-grade. The commonest are *small cell (neuroendocrine) carcinomas* which are high-grade tumours showing a diffuse growth pattern of basaloid 'blue' cells with scanty cytoplasm and nuclear atypia with nuclear moulding, a 'salt and pepper, chromatin pattern and numerous mitotic figures. These are often bulky and locally advanced at presentation.

2.2   Endometrium

The majority of endometrial carcinomas are oestrogen driven and preceded by hyperplasia, the remainder being oestrogen independent (Table 2.2). These are broadly divided into types 1 and 2 to reflect their different behaviour (Table 2.3). These may show diffuse thickening or a localised mass, which may be polypoidal, with variable myometrial invasion.

Table 2.2 WHO classification of carcinomas of epithelial tumours of the uterine corpus

WHO classification of carcinomas of the endometrium
Endometrioid
Usual type
Squamous differentiation
Villoglandular
Secretory
Mucinous
Clear cell carcinoma
Serous
Neuroendocrine
Low grade (carcinoid)
High grade (large cell, small cell)
Mixed cell adenocarcinoma
Undifferentiated
Dedifferentiated

Table 2.3 Differences between type 1 and type 2 endometrial cancers

Contrasting type 1 and type 2 endometrial carcinomas	Type 1 endometrial adenocarcinoma	Type 2 endometrial adenocarcinoma
Histological types	Endometrioid, adenosquamous, mucinous	Serous, clear cell, carcinosarcoma
Proportion of endometrial carcinomas	70–80%	20–30%
Behaviour	Indolent	Aggressive
Age group	Perimenopausal	Postmenopausal
Aetiology	Related to unopposed oestrogen exposure	No relation to oestrogen exposure
Grade	1–3, generally lower grade	High-grade nuclear features
Prognosis	Good	Poor

Architecturally, *endometrioid carcinoma* comprises closely packed or coalescing glands lined by columnar cells resulting in smooth luminal contours (Fig. 2.3). Grading (Table 2.4) is defined by the extent of non-squamous solid growth and, to a lesser degree, by nuclear atypia, as this broadly follows the architectural grade. Low-grade architecture with high-grade nuclear features should not be seen in endometrioid carcinoma, and an alternative diagnosis, e.g. serous carcinoma, should be entertained. There is immunoreactivity for oestrogen and progesterone receptor. *Squamous differentiation* is commonly seen; it is not included in the assessment of solid architecture for grading. *Mucinous carcinomas* are low-grade tumours composed of mucin-containing columnar cells arranged in glandular or villoglandular patterns. Morphology can be confused with endocervical carcinoma, and immunohistochemistry can be used to distinguish them. *Serous carcinomas* are typically composed of complex papillae, but glandular architecture is also seen. They are distinguished from endometrioid carcinoma by their high-grade nuclear atypia; they are generally ER and PR negative and show aberrant p53 expression. *Clear cell carcinoma* possesses cells with clear or eosinophilic cytoplasm arranged in papillary, tubulocystic or solid patterns. *Neuroendocrine tumours* of the endometrium are rare; these are exophytic,

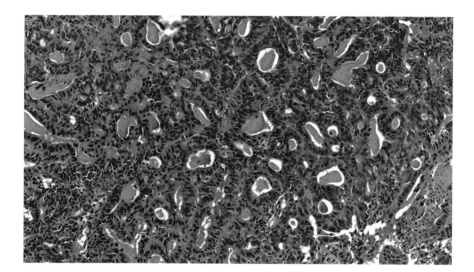

Fig. 2.3 Endometrioid grade 1 adenocarcinoma composed of glands arranged back to back with smooth luminal edges

Table 2.4 FIGO grading of endometrioid carcinoma

Architectural grading of endometrioid carcinoma	
Grade 1[a]	<5 % of tumour comprises non-squamous solid areas
Grade 2[a]	6–50 % of tumour comprises non-squamous solid areas
Grade 3	>50 % of tumour comprises non-squamous solid areas

[a]The presence of grade 3 nuclei involving >50 % of the tumour justifies upgrading by one grade

polypoid tumours with nested, solid or cribriform architecture. Nuclear features are similar to neuroendocrine tumours elsewhere in the body. *Mixed carcinomas* are defined by being composed of two histological types of carcinoma, one of which must be type 2. *Undifferentiated carcinoma* is a malignant epithelial neoplasm with no differentiation, often occurring as a large polypoidal mass. *Dedifferentiated carcinoma* is a combination of undifferentiated carcinoma with grade 1–2 endometrioid carcinoma. *Carcinosarcoma* is included here as it is believed to be epithelial in derivation with sarcomatous transformation occurring through epithelial-mesenchymal transition; these show an intimate admixture of high-grade epithelial and mesenchymal (sarcomatous) components in highly variable proportions.

2.3   Ovary

Ovarian malignancies can be of epithelial, sex cord-stromal or germ cell origin. Epithelial malignancies account for 95 % of tumours; the commonest of these is high-grade serous carcinoma, which is believed to arise from the fimbrial end of the fallopian tube in the majority of cases.

WHO classification of malignant ovarian tumours
Epithelial
High-grade serous
Endometrioid
Clear cell
Mucinous
Low-grade serous
Brenner
Seromucinous
Undifferentiated
Germ cell
Dysgerminoma
Yolk sac tumour
Embryonal carcinoma
Choriocarcinoma
Mature teratoma
Immature teratoma
Mixed germ cell tumour
Sex cord-stromal
Adult granulosa cell tumour
Juvenile granulosa cell tumour
Others
Mesothelioma
Lymphoma
Secondary deposits

Epithelial neoplasms are termed 'benign', 'borderline' or 'malignant' and may present as solid or cystic lesions. *Borderline tumours* possess features intermediate between benign and malignant counterparts. Typically there is epithelial stratification and formation of papillary excrescences with mildly atypical cells. There is no stromal invasion. Cells may be shed from the surface of the tumour to involve any peritoneal surface in the pelvis forming 'implants'. Thorough sampling is undertaken (one block/1 cm of tumour maximum diameter) to avoid the possibility of a malignant tumour being missed.

High-grade serous carcinomas are lined by markedly atypical cells arranged in papillae with discohesive cells falling away from the tips (Fig. 2.4). Stromal invasion presents as fused glands with characteristic slit-like spaces. Psammomatous calcification is frequently seen. Currently the majority of high-grade serous carcinomas are believed to arise from tubal epithelium, manifesting in practice as gross or microscopic involvement of the fimbrial end; distal tubal involvement may be evident on imaging. *Low-grade serous carcinomas* have a variety of architectural patterns and a uniform population of cells with relatively monomorphic nuclei. Psammomatous calcification is typically widespread. *Mucinous carcinomas* are cystic lesions containing viscid mucin. The lining epithelium is usually of gastrointestinal type (i.e. resembling stomach mucosa) but may also recapitulate endocervical-type epithelium. *Endometrioid carcinomas* are identical to those arising from the endometrium. It may be difficult to distinguish synchronous endometrioid carcinomas of the ovary and endometrium from disease in one organ metastasizing to other organs. Distinction is important as the latter scenario affords a worse prognosis. *Clear cell carcinoma* often develops in a background of endometriosis; this can present with solid, tubulocystic or papillary patterns. Cells can either have clear or eosinophilic cytoplasm with a 'hobnail' luminal profile (Fig. 2.5). *Malignant*

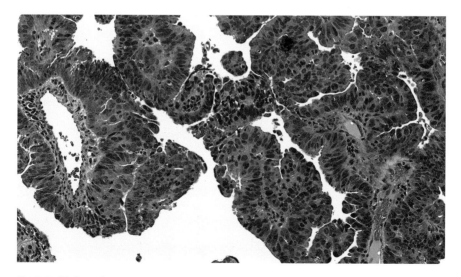

Fig. 2.4 High-grade serous carcinomas showing papillary architecture and marked nuclear atypia

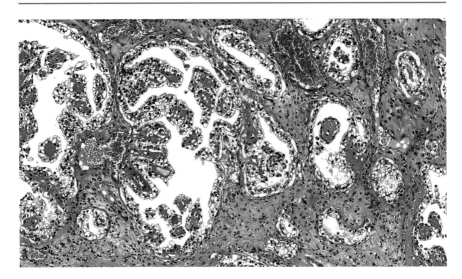

Fig. 2.5 Clear cell carcinoma composed of cells with optically clear cytoplasm and distinct cell outlines forming glands and papillae

Brenner tumour is the eponymous name given to neoplasms consisting of transitional epithelium, resembling invasive urothelial carcinoma. *Seromucinous tumours* comprise serous and endocervical-type mucinous epithelium.

Germ cell tumours and *sex cord-stromal* tumours are rare tumours usually managed in the UK by specialist centres. In general, they show similar features to those seen in the testis.

Key Points

Cervix

Carcinomas of the cervix are exophytic (polypoidal/papillary), ulcerative or endophytic.

Squamous cell carcinoma (SCC) shows sheets or nests of polygonal, squamous cells invading the underlying cervical stroma.

Adenocarcinoma is a malignancy of glandular mucosa which is usually associated with HPV.

Endometrium

The majority of endometrial carcinomas are oestrogen driven.

Grading is defined by the extent of non-squamous solid growth and, to a lesser degree, by nuclear atypia.

Ovary

Ovarian malignancies can be of epithelial, sex cord-stromal or germ cell origin.

Epithelial malignancies account for 95 % of tumours; the commonest of these is high-grade serous carcinoma, which often arises in the distal fallopian tube.

Further Reading

1. Kurman RJ, Ellenson LH, Ronnett BM, editors. Blaustein's pathology of the female genital tract. 6th ed. New York: Springer; 2011.
2. Kurman RJ, Carcangiu ML, Herrington CS, Young RH, editors. WHO classification of tumours of female reproductive organs. 4th ed. Lyon: IARC; 2014.
3. Robboy SJ, Mutter GL, Prat J, Bentley RC, Russell P, Anderson MC, editors. Robboy's pathology of the female reproductive tract. 2nd ed. London: Churchill Livingstone; 2009.

An Overview of the Management of Gynaecological Cancers

3

Nicholas Reed and Azmat Sadozye

Contents

3.1   Cervical Cancer

3.1.1   Management of Primary Cervical Cancer

The management of microinvasive disease is usually by localised excision either by laser loop excision (LLETZ), cold cautery or cone biopsy, with careful and regular follow-up in colposcopy clinics as a small proportion will develop recurrent disease requiring intervention. More commonly patients will have invasive disease, and following the results of the staging procedures that have been described in Chaps. 1 and 4 and after discussion at the MDT or tumour board, clinical management will be decided. For early disease in younger patients, tumours less than 4 cm, surgery consisting of radical hysterectomy and lymph node dissection is the treatment of

N. Reed (✉) • A. Sadozye
Department of Clinical Oncology, Beatson Oncology Centre, Gartnavel General Hospital, Glasgow, Scotland
e-mail: nick.reed@ggc.scot.nhs.uk; azmat.sadozye@ggc.scot.nhs.uk

© Springer International Publishing Switzerland 2016
T. Barwick, A. Rockall (eds.), *PET/CT in Gynecological Cancers*,
Clinicians' Guides to Radionuclide Hybrid Imaging, DOI 10.1007/978-3-319-29249-6_3

choice. Increasingly the laparoscopic approach is being used with its faster recovery times. These approaches are summarised in Table 3.1. Trachelectomy, a fertility-sparing surgery, is only used selectively in localised tumours less than 2 cm in size. Suitability for trachelectomy is determined by clinical examination and pelvic MRI (Chap. 4).

For patients with tumours larger than 4 cm or in older patients or those unfit for surgery who have smaller volume disease, concomitant chemoradiation remains the gold standard. Five important clinical trials were published in 2000 followed by a consensus statement from the National Cancer Institute which recommended that concurrent chemotherapy (usually, weekly cisplatin at 40 mg/m^2) should be given along with full pelvic radiation and intracavitary brachytherapy [4]. The use of intensity-modulated radiation therapy (IMRT) is increasingly being adopted as a standard of care and should allow reductions in toxicity and offers the potential to escalate the dose. Other approaches include the use of induction chemotherapy prior to chemoradiation and the use of maintenance or consolidation treatment with chemotherapy following treatment. These are not yet standard care but are currently being investigated in important international clinical trials.

Following surgery, there will be discussions on the need for adjuvant treatment. The Gynaecological Oncology Group (GOG) trials of adjuvant treatment have identified risk factors which usually include factors such as tumour size, more than 50 % stromal infiltration, parametrial extension, lymphovascular space invasion, grade III pathology and positive nodes [7]. When at least one of these factors is present, adjuvant concomitant chemoradiation will be advised with weekly cisplatin and full pelvic radiation followed by vaginal brachytherapy. These are summarised in Table 3.2.

For those presenting as stage IVb, chemotherapy would normally be the treatment of choice with platinum-based regimes, whilst palliative radiation may be

Table 3.1 Summary of treatment options for cervical cancer

Disease stage	Treatment options
Microinvasive disease	Loop excision (LLETZ)
	Cone biopsy
Early invasive disease <4 cm	Radical hysterectomy
	Lymph node dissection
Locally advanced disease >4 cm	Chemoradiation and brachytherapy
Metastatic or relapsed disease	Chemotherapy
	Palliative radiation

Table 3.2 Risk factors for disease relapse in cervical cancers

Risk factors for relapse (modified from GOG)
Grade 3 histology
Parametrial disease
>50 stromal invasion
Lymphovascular space invasion
Positive nodes
Tumours >3 cm

used to control symptoms such as pain or bleeding. Cisplatin (or carboplatin) and paclitaxel are generally accepted to be the most effective treatments. In some unfit elderly patients presenting with very advanced disease, a single fraction of radiotherapy of 10 Gy may be valuable to stop bleeding and may be repeated.

3.1.2 Management of Recurrent Cervical Cancer

The management of recurrent disease will usually be determined by prior treatment; so for those who underwent prior surgery, chemoradiation will be offered. If however the patient has had prior radiation and disease is confined to the pelvis, consideration may be given to exenterative procedures with or without chemotherapy. The laterally extended endopelvic resection (LEER) is increasingly being adopted for use in these circumstances. PET/CT is essential in staging these patients prior to such radical procedures (Chap. 7). A number of chemotherapy trials have shown that cisplatin and paclitaxel are two of the best drugs, and a recent trial has shown improved survival from the addition of bevacizumab to this combination [10]. When patients relapse, it is important to involve palliative care teams for symptom control.

3.2 Uterine Cancer

3.2.1 Management of Primary Uterine Cancer

Uterine cancer is generally a surgically treated disease [2]. Most patients are suitable for hysterectomy, but in our society, with ever-increasing levels of obesity, patients with very high BMIs may be turned down. The majority of patients have low- or intermediate-risk disease (imaging showing disease involving inner half and biopsy showing grade I or grade II histological tumours) and require a simple hysterectomy, bilateral salpingo-oophorectomy and washings (Table 3.3). Two major clinical trials have failed to show any survival advantage to pelvic and/or para-aortic lymphadenectomy. Nevertheless, there remain advocates of lymphadenectomy for staging purposes, which may help to tailor subsequent treatment. The case for lymphadenectomy may be stronger for grade III tumours, uterine carcinosarcomas, clear cell and serous cancers when there are higher rates of lymph node involvement. Thus pelvic and para-aortic lymphadenectomy will be recommended providing there are no contraindications to this approach such as obesity, cardiovascular disease, diabetes and hypertension.

Table 3.3 Risk factors for endometrial cancer

Lower-risk groups	Higher-risk groups
Age 60 or less	Age over 60
Grades 1 and 2	Grade 3
Inner half myometrial invasion	Outer half myometrial invasion
Lymphovascular space invasion	

Table 3.4 Prognostic groups requiring adjuvant therapy in endometrial cancer

Grade vs stage to assign risk groups in endometrial cancer			
	Grade 1	Grade 2	Grade 3
Stage 1A	Low	Low	Intermediate
Stage 1B	Intermediate	Intermediate	High

Adjuvant treatment will then be determined by the findings of the risk factors from the pathology. Age over 60, outer half myometrial involvement and grade III tumours (serous and clear cell and uterine carcinosarcomas) indicate a worse prognosis. Traditionally adjuvant radiotherapy [6] was given to all intermediate- or high-risk cases; these are shown in Table 3.4. However, several clinical trials have shown that adjuvant radiotherapy probably has no impact on overall survival despite improving local control. A subsequent trial comparing vaginal brachytherapy and external beam radiotherapy in the low/intermediate-risk groups has shown no survival advantage to external beam radiotherapy, so increasingly vaginal brachytherapy alone is used in these patients. The use of chemotherapy is controversial, but many feel that for G3 tumours (or high-risk histologies such as clear cell, serous and carcinosarcomas), particularly when lymphovascular space invasion is present, the risk of metastatic disease is significantly higher and that adjuvant carboplatin and paclitaxel may improve survival.

For patients with inoperable disease (usually for medical reasons), the use of radiotherapy alone may be considered. In selective patients, 5-year survivals of up to 60% may be achieved. This would normally require a full course of external beam radiotherapy together with some form of intracavitary boost. This is inferior to what would be expected with surgery alone but avoids the significant risk of morbidity and mortality in these high-risk patients.

3.2.2 Management of Recurrent Disease

Patients with G3 tumours especially serous and clear cell have a higher risk of early recurrence, whereas the risk of recurrence in the low- and intermediate-risk patients is relatively low. When these lower-risk tumours recur, there is often a longer disease-free interval, and they are more likely to be oestrogen and progestogen receptor positive in which case hormonal therapy with tamoxifen, megestrol acetate or an aromatase inhibitor may be prescribed. Between 20 and 40%, response rates will be seen under these circumstances with some long-term survivors. For patients with early relapsing disease usually with high-risk features, chemotherapy is the treatment of choice, and carboplatin and paclitaxel are identified as the two most active drugs. For patients with relapse, doxorubicin-based regimes may be considered, but results are often disappointing [3]. A number of molecular markers have been identified in endometrial cancers, and loss of pTEN and changes in the mTOR and PI3 kinase pathways may be demonstrated. Modest responses have been seen with drugs that work through these pathways, but rather disappointingly the molecular markers and clinical response do not always correlate (Table 3.5).

Table 3.5 Higher-risk endometrial cancers

High-risk endometrial cancers
Serous endometrial cancers
Clear cell cancers
Carcinosarcomas
Mixed tumours

3.3 Ovarian Cancer

Ovarian cancer is primarily a surgically treated disease [5]. The standard surgical approach is full comprehensive staging with total hysterectomy, bilateral salpingo-oophorectomy, omentectomy, blind biopsies and lymphadenectomy with attempts to achieve complete debulking (i.e. no residual disease). In nearly all cases, chemotherapy is given afterwards. However, for stage IVb patients with extensive liver, splenic or extra-abdominal metastases and for patients with stage IIIc disease with bulky supracolic disease, neoadjuvant chemotherapy with delayed surgery may be considered as an alternative. Two recent trials from Europe, EORTC 55971 and CHORUS, have shown that in patients with bulky disease unlikely to be optimally resectable, the use of neoadjuvant (up front) chemotherapy leads to a higher rate of achieving optimal surgical cytoreduction [11]. Survival was not inferior and recovery time and morbidity were reduced. Perhaps more controversial is the management of primary peritoneal tumours where there is no bulky disease in the ovaries. Some would argue that in these patients, chemotherapy alone may be considered, but this has not yet been subjected to clinical trial. New molecular markers have identified five subtypes (Table 3.6) with some of the commonly associated markers which may help to personalise treatments [1].

Following surgery virtually all patients will be advised to receive adjuvant chemotherapy. The exceptions may be for optimally staged 1a, G1/G2 tumours where it may be possible to withhold chemotherapy with fully informed consent. For all other cases, chemotherapy is advised assuming the patient is fit enough. The standard therapy is a combination of carboplatin with paclitaxel, and increasingly, particularly for patients with residual disease, adjuvant bevacizumab has been shown to improve progression-free survival [8]. There is some controversy as to whether this should be used at the time of initial treatment or for recurrence, but either way, the use of adjuvant bevacizumab has become a practice. Intraperitoneal chemotherapy may also be considered especially for patients who have achieved optimal cytoreduction where significant survival benefit has been demonstrated. A variety of other molecular-targeted agents are being investigated, and we can expect to see these incorporated into clinical management [1].

The treatment of recurrent disease will be determined by a number of factors, most important of which is the treatment-free interval. This is shown in Table 3.7. Responses to platinum in this resistant or refractory settings are generally less than 10 %. Disease relapsing beyond 6 months is recognised as platinum sensitive, but there is a transition period where the interval lies between 6 and 12 months known as partially platinum sensitive. In this setting, there is much more controversy about

Table 3.6 Subtypes of ovarian cancer and mutations

Histological type	Mutations isolated
Serous: high grade	*TP53*
Serous: low grade	BRAF, KRAS
Endometrioid	pTEN, BRAF, KRAS
	beta-catenin, PI3 kinase
Clear cell	ARID1a
Mucinous	KRAS
Carcinosarcoma	Non-specific but includes p53

Table 3.7 Treatment of recurrent ovarian cancer as determined by treatment-free interval

	Response to platinum	
	Time to recurrence (months)	Response to further platinum
Platinum sensitive Relapse after 12 months	>12	30–60%
Partially platinum sensitive Relapse between 6 and 12 months	6–12	25–30%
Platinum resistant Relapse within 6 months	<6	<10%
Platinum refractory Do not respond to platinum	No initial response	N/A

the regime, but a recent trial has shown that liposomal doxorubicin and trabectedin have a superior effect. For patients relapsing beyond 12 months, it would be normal to consider treatment with a platinum-based regime. Traditionally carboplatin and paclitaxel but alternatively carboplatin and liposomal doxorubicin or carboplatin and gemcitabine will be used. Again the use of targeted agents in these settings is increasingly being adopted. These include bevacizumab and cediranib, but it is anticipated that others will become adopted over the next 5 years.

Increasingly patients with recurrent ovarian cancer will be re-challenged with treatments, some receiving three, four, five or more lines, and patients may survive a number of years. For patients with BRCA mutation, the PARP inhibitors are showing exciting activity. Testing younger patients with serous cancer is becoming standard [9].

Key Points
Cervical Cancer
The management of microinvasive disease is usually by localised excision and regular follow-up in colposcopy clinics.
In early disease in younger patients, tumours less than 4 cm, radical hysterectomy and lymph node dissection are the treatment of choice.

In patients with tumours larger than 4 cm or in older patients or those unfit for surgery who have smaller volume disease, concomitant chemoradiation remains the gold standard.

The management of recurrent disease will usually be determined by prior treatment.

Uterine Cancer

Uterine cancer is generally a surgically treatable disease.

Majority of patients with low- or intermediate-risk disease require a simple hysterectomy, bilateral salpingo-oophorectomy and washings.

In patients with inoperable disease, radiotherapy alone may be considered.

Patients with G3 tumours especially serous and clear cell have a higher risk of early recurrence.

Ovarian Cancer

The standard surgical approach is full comprehensive staging with total hysterectomy, bilateral salpingo-oophorectomy, omentectomy, blind biopsies and lymphadenectomy with attempts to achieve complete debulking.

Following surgery, virtually all patients will be advised to receive adjuvant chemotherapy (exceptions: optimally staged 1a, G1/G2 tumours where it may be possible to withhold chemotherapy with fully informed consent).

The treatment of recurrent disease will be determined by a number of factors, most important of which is the treatment-free interval.

References

1. Despierre E, Yesilyurt BT, Lambrechts S, Johnson N, Verheijen R, van der Burg M, Casado A, Rustin G, Berns E, Leunen K, Amant F, Moerman P, Lambrechts D. Epithelial ovarian cancer: rationale for changing the one-fits-all standard treatment regimen to subtype-specific treatment. Vergote I; EORTC GCG and EORTC GCG translational research group. Int J Gynecol Cancer. 2014;24(3):468–77.
2. Falcone F, Balbi G, Di Martino L, Grauso F, Salzillo ME, Messalli EM. Surgical management of early endometrial cancer: an update and proposal of a therapeutic algorithm. Med Sci Monit. 2014;20:1298–313.
3. Fleming GF. Systemic chemotherapy for uterine carcinoma: metastatic and adjuvant. J Clin Oncol. 2007;25(20):2983–90.
4. Gaffney DK. Optimal therapy for IB2 and IIA2 cervical cancer: surgery or chemoradiotherapy? J Gynecol Oncol. 2012;23(4):207–9.
5. Goff BA. Advanced ovarian cancer: what should be the standard of care? J Gynecol Oncol. 2013;24(1):83–91.
6. Klopp A, Smith BD, Alektiar K, Cabrera A, Damato AL, Erickson B, Fleming G, Gaffney D, Greven K, Lu K, Miller D, Moore D, Petereit D, Schefter T, Small Jr W, Yashar C, Viswanathan AN. The role of postoperative radiation therapy for endometrial cancer: executive summary of an American Society for Radiation Oncology evidence-based guideline. Pract Radiat Oncol. 2014;4(3):137–44.

7. Monk BJ, Tian C, Rose PG, Lanciano R. Which clinical/pathologic factors matter in the era of chemoradiation as treatment for locally advanced cervical carcinoma? Analysis of two Gynecologic Oncology Group (GOG) trials. Gynecol Oncol. 2007;105(2):427–33.
8. Monk BJ, Pujade-Lauraine E, Burger RA. Integrating bevacizumab into the management of epithelial ovarian cancer: the controversy of front-line versus recurrent disease. Ann Oncol. 2013;24 Suppl 10:x53–8.
9. Pennington KP, Swisher EM. Hereditary ovarian cancer: beyond the usual suspects. Gynecol Oncol. 2012;124(2):347–53.
10. Tewari KS, Sill MW, Long 3rd HJ, Penson RT, Huang H, Ramondetta LM, Landrum LM, Oaknin A, Reid TJ, Leitao MM, Michael HE, Monk BJ. Improved survival with bevacizumab in advanced cervical cancer. N Engl J Med. 2014;370(8):734–43.
11. Vergote I, Amant F, Kristensen G, Ehlen T, Reed NS, Casado A. Primary surgery or neoadjuvant chemotherapy followed by interval debulking surgery in advanced ovarian cancer. Eur J Cancer. 2011;47 Suppl 3:S88–92.

Radiological Imaging in Gynaecological Malignancies

4

Nishat Bharwani and Victoria Stewart

Contents

N. Bharwani (✉)
Department of Surgery & Cancer, Imperial College, London, UK

Department of Imaging, St Mary's Hospital, Imperial College Healthcare NHS Trust,
London, UK
e-mail: nishat.bharwani@imperial.nhs.uk

V. Stewart
Department of Radiology, Imperial College Healthcare NHS Trust,
Charing Cross Hospital, London, UK
e-mail: victoria.stewart@imperial.nhs.uk

© Springer International Publishing Switzerland 2016
T. Barwick, A. Rockall (eds.), *PET/CT in Gynecological Cancers*,
Clinicians' Guides to Radionuclide Hybrid Imaging, DOI 10.1007/978-3-319-29249-6_4

4.1   Normal Anatomy

The uterus is divided into three anatomical regions: the fundus, body (uterine corpus) and cervix. The body is formed of three layers: the endometrium (inner lining), myometrium (muscular wall) and serosa (outer surface). There are physiological variations in the imaging appearances of these layers depending on hormonal status and age. The myometrium is divided into the junctional zone (JZ or inner myometrium) which lies adjacent to the endometrium and the outer myometrium. The cervix also demonstrates three layers which are in continuity with the layers of the uterine body: the inner endocervical canal and two layers which make up the cervical stroma and are continuous with the layers of the myometrium.

The normal appearance of the ovaries also varies with hormonal status and age. In premenopausal patients, an ovary has a volume of 5–14 ml and contains numerous (5–15) follicles depending on the phase of menstruation. After the menopause the ovaries atrophy and there is no follicular function.

4.2   Imaging Modalities and Technique

FIGO staging is a clinical (cervix) or surgical-pathological (endometrial and ovarian) staging system, and imaging findings do not change this. However, imaging has an important role in treatment planning and evaluation of complications [13].

Ultrasound (US) and magnetic resonance imaging (MRI) are the imaging modalities of choice for detailed investigation of the female pelvis. Normal US and MRI appearances of the female reproductive system are shown in Fig. 4.1.

Pelvic MRI may be performed on a 1.5 or 3 T system ideally using a multichannel pelvic phased-array coil. The patient is fasted for 4–6 h and imaged with a partially filled bladder following administration of an antiperistaltic agent.

Contrast-enhanced CT (CECT) plays an important role in the identification of disease beyond the uterus and ovaries, allowing evaluation of the peritoneal surfaces, omentum, upper abdominal viscera, thorax and nodal stations. Water taken orally 1 h prior to the scan provides negative contrast within the small bowel lumen and can help demonstrate peritoneal disease.

4.3   Cervical Cancer

4.3.1   Primary Diagnosis/Staging

Patients with cervical cancer usually present for imaging when a diagnosis of invasive cancer has been made histologically. MRI is the optimal imaging modality for pretreatment local staging of cervical cancer.

The most important sequences are high-resolution sagittal T2-weighted (T2W) series and an axial oblique T2W sequence orientated perpendicular to the long axis of the cervix (see full MRI protocol in Table 4.1). MRI should be performed at least 7–10 days after biopsy [9] to reduce post-biopsy artefact which can cause difficulties with MR evaluation of tumour extent.

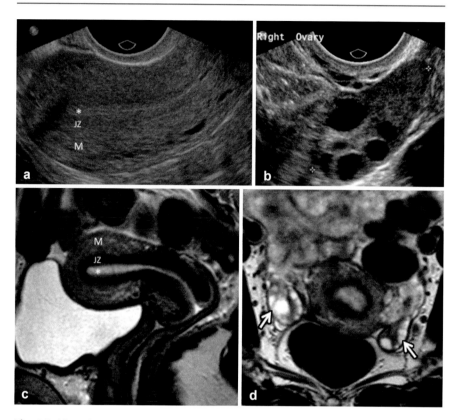

Fig. 4.1 Normal premenopausal appearances of the uterus and ovaries on ultrasound (**a**, **b**) and MRI (**c**, **d**). Images show two different patients with anteverted, anteflexed uteri (**a**, **c**) showing clearly defined zonal anatomy (* - endometrial complex; *JZ* – junctional zone or inner myometrium; *M* – outer myometrium) which continue into the uterine cervix. The ovaries show typical appearances with several simple follicles both on US (**b**) and MRI (**d** – *white arrows*))

Table 4.1 Recommended sequences for staging MRI in cervical cancer

Sequence	Plane	Reason
T1W and T2W (renal hila to the symphysis pubis)	Axial (large FOV)	Evaluate para-aortic LN Assess for hydronephrosis Bone marrow (T1W)
T2W	Sagittal	Visualise tumour extent and measure size Assess for extension into the uterus, vagina, bladder and rectum
T2W	Axial oblique (small FOV, high resolution perpendicular to the endocervical canal)	Measure tumour size Assessment of parametrial and pelvic sidewall invasion Nodal evaluation
DWI (as LFOV T1W/T2W)	Axial	Assessment of tumour and LN

T1W T1-weighted, *T2W* T2-weighted, *DWI* diffusion-weighted imaging, *FOV* field of view, *LN* lymph node

Table 4.2 Selection criteria for trachelectomy

Clinical/pathological	Imaging
Desire to preserve fertility	FIGO stage IA or IB
Confirmed diagnosis of cervical cancer, especially squamous, adenocarcinoma or adenosquamous carcinoma	Tumour size ≤2 cm
Limited endocervical involvement at colposcopy	No lymph node involvement
	Estimated length of remaining cervix ≥1 cm
	No stromal invasion more than 1 cm

CECT of the chest, abdomen and pelvis is indicated in patients with advanced disease.

Patients with cervical cancer have two main treatment options – surgery and primary chemoradiotherapy (CRT) (Chap. 3). The role of pretreatment imaging is to help determine which is most appropriate.

Stage I disease: Tumour confined to the cervix.
Stage IA tumours are only visible microscopically, while stage IB and above are clinically visible (see FIGO staging in Table 1.1 of Chap. 1). The size of the tumour has prognostic implications; tumour volume also has prognostic implications; however, this parameter does not contribute to the FIGO stage.
Cervical cancer is intermediate to high signal intensity (SI) on T2W images compared to the normal low T2W SI of cervical stroma. The presence of an intact low T2W ring of cervical stroma around the tumour has a high negative predictive value for parametrial invasion [6].
Trachelectomy (vaginal or abdominal) can be considered in women with organ-confined disease who meet certain criteria (Table 4.2) and wish to preserve fertility.
Stage II disease: Tumour invades beyond the uterus, but not to the pelvic wall or lower vagina.
If an exophytic tumour expands the vagina but does not disrupt the normal low T2W SI of the vaginal wall, it is still confined to the cervix. However, if there is disruption of the low T2W SI in the upper two thirds of the vaginal wall, then the tumour is upstaged to IIA. The parametrium is a band of connective tissue that extends out laterally from the supravaginal cervix between the layers of the broad ligament. When parametrial extension is present, the low SI of the cervical stroma is disrupted, and there is an irregular infiltrating margin between the tumour and the parametrium (stage IIB).
Stage III disease: Tumour extends to the pelvic wall and/or involves the lower vagina.
When tumour extends to involve the lower third of the vagina, then it is considered stage IIIA.

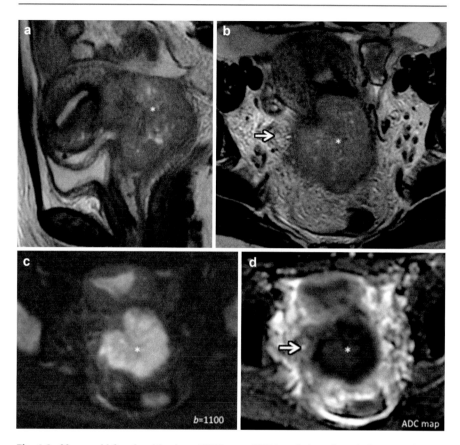

Fig. 4.2 32 year old female with a large FIGO stage IIIB barrel-shaped cervical tumour. Sagittal (**a**) and high resolution axial (**b**) T2-weighted MR images demonstrate a bulky predominantly intermediate T2W signal intensity tumour (*) with right parametrial invasion and right pelvic side wall involvement with a right hydronephrosis (*white arrow*). Diffusion weighted images, $b = 1000$ s/mm² (**c**) and corresponding apparent diffusion coefficient (ADC) map (**d**), show significant restriction of diffusivity suggesting high cellularity in keeping with cervical cancer

Often the first imaging sign of pelvic sidewall involvement is the presence of hydronephrosis due to obstruction of the ureter(s) which lie immediately deep to the peritoneum (stage IIIB, Fig. 4.2).

Stage IV: Tumour extends beyond the true pelvis or involves the mucosa of the bladder or rectum (biopsy proven).

MRI can accurately assess tumour invasion into adjacent structures, and loss of the normal low T2W SI of the bladder/bowel wall is a sign of early invasion. Early involvement of the wall is important to document as it can be a potential site for complications (e.g. fistula formation) at a later stage. However, the tumour is only upstaged to stage IVA if tumour extends to involve the mucosa.

Nodal status.

Nodal involvement is not part of FIGO staging, but it has significant management and prognostic implications and is the single strongest predictor of long-term survival [4, 8]. Nodal spread can often be distant in cervical cancer.

4.3.2 Follow-Up

In patients treated with CRT, serial MRI can be used to monitor response.

Approximately one third of patients will recur within 3 years of their primary treatment [2]. Recurrence is usually central, involving the vaginal vault following surgery or within the cervix post-CRT; however, distant relapse can also be seen involving the liver/lungs or within the retroperitoneal lymph nodes above the radiation field [1].

4.3.3 Limitations/Pitfalls of MRI

- In the presence of a small tumour, post-biopsy changes can sometimes make interpretation difficult.
- Early parametrial extension can be difficult to identify, and complete loss of the low signal cervical ring does not always indicate definite parametrial extension. Evaluation under anaesthesia (EUA) combined with MRI is often the best way to determine appropriate management.
- In some cases it can be difficult to ascertain if a tumour involving the lower endometrium and cervical canal is a primary cervical tumour with uterine involvement or vice versa. In these cases histopathological assessment and immunohistochemistry can help.

4.4 Endometrial Cancer

4.4.1 Primary Diagnosis/Staging

4.4.1.1 Ultrasound

When endometrial cancer is suspected clinically, transvaginal ultrasound is the optimal method to demonstrate the endometrial cavity. Endometrial thickening or irregularity is suspicious particularly if there is increased vascularity. In postmenopausal patients, an endometrial thickness of over 5 mm is considered abnormal and requires endometrial sampling [3].

4.4.1.2 MRI

Once a histopathological diagnosis of malignancy has been established, local staging may be undertaken with MRI, and routine pelvic sequences are found in Table 4.3. The most important sequences are a sagittal T2W and a high-resolution axial oblique sequence orientated perpendicular to the endometrial cavity, to assess for myometrial invasion. Dynamic contrast-enhanced acquisitions are helpful in

Table 4.3 Recommended MRI sequences for staging in endometrial cancer

Sequence	Plane	Reason
T1W and T2W (renal hila to the symphysis pubis)	Axial (large FOV)	Evaluate para-aortic LN Bone marrow (T1W)
T2W	Sagittal	Visualise tumour extent and degree of myometrial invasion Assess for serosal extension and involvement of the uterus, vagina, bladder and rectum
T2W	Axial oblique (small FOV, high resolution perpendicular to the endometrial cavity)	Assessment of myometrial extension and size of the uterus Nodal evaluation
DWI (as for T2W)	Axial oblique and sagittal	Assessment of tumour and LN
3D dynamic contrast acquisition with T1W fat saturation	Sagittal	Assessment of myometrial invasion; reformat in oblique axial plane

T1W T1-weighted, *T2W* T2-weighted, *DWI* diffusion-weighted imaging, *FOV* field of view, *LN* lymph node

determining the depth of myometrial invasion, and there is an increasing use of diffusion-weighted imaging (DWI).

As the surgical management for endometrial cancer is hysterectomy, in all but advanced disease, it is helpful to comment on the size of the uterus, as this may dictate the surgical approach (laparoscopic versus open).

Stage I disease: Tumour is confined to the uterus.
The tumour usually manifests as an area of intermediate T2W SI within the high-
 signal endometrial cavity.
Myometrial invasion is suspected if the tumour breaches the low T2W SI junctional
 zone which surrounds the endometrium. Tumour invasion of less than 50 % of
 myometrial thickness is stage IA (Fig. 4.3), and invasion over 50 % upstages to
 IB. The surgical management is altered for higher-grade IB tumours which
 require nodal resection for accurate FIGO staging, as the incidence of lymph
 node involvement is increased.
Most studies have reported increased accuracy in assessing the depth of invasion
 when dynamic contrast acquisition sequences are used [7, 12]. Small tumours
 enhance faster than the endometrium which can help in small cancer detection,
 whereas invasive tumours enhance less than the surrounding normal myometrium. High-resolution DWI may also improve the confidence of the radiologist
 in accurately diagnosing the depth of myometrial invasion [10].
Stage II disease: Tumour involves the cervix.
Cervical stromal involvement is an important distinction as it is treated with radical
 rather than simple hysterectomy. Tumours that extend into the endocervical
 canal but not into the stroma remain stage I. Normal cervical stroma is typically
 low in T2W SI and when involved becomes invaded by the intermediate T2W SI
 tumour.

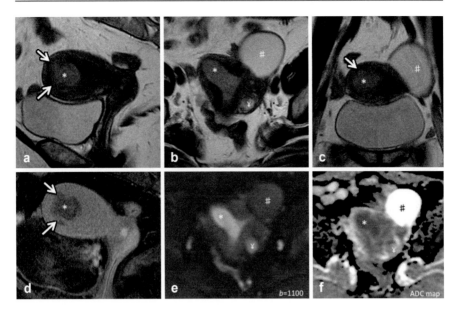

Fig. 4.3 56 year old female presenting with post-menopausal bleeding and biopsy-proven endometrial carcinoma. Sagittal (**a**), axial (**b**) and high resolution axial oblique (**c**) T2-weighted imaging demonstrate an intermediate signal intensity mass distending the endometrial cavity (*) predominantly extending into the right cornua and invading the myometrium to less than 50 % of it's thickness (*white arrows*) in keeping with a FIGO stage IA tumour. Note that the myometrium in the right cornua is thinned by the large tumour in the cavity which makes assessment of depth of invasion more difficult. Dynamic contrast-enhanced MR image (**d**) acquired at 60 seconds post-contrast administration clearly depicts the endometrial tumour enhancing to a lesser degree than the adjacent normal myometrium (*) and an irregular endometrial-myometrial interface in keeping with myometrial invasion (*white arrows*). Diffusion weighted images, $b = 1000$ s/mm^2 (**e**) and corresponding apparent diffusion coefficient (ADC) map (**f**), show significant restriction of diffusivity (*) suggesting high cellularity and in keeping with endometrial cancer. Incidental note is made of a simple left ovarian cyst (♯) and celluar leiomeyoma (¥)

Stage III disease: Tumour extension beyond uterus.

If the tumour extends beyond the cervix to the parametrium (IIIB), the dark ring of cervical stroma becomes breached and irregular. It is crucial to have good high-resolution axial images of the cervix to evaluate this, and if tangential images are not performed and orientation to the uterine body is different, then evaluation may be difficult.

When tumour extends beyond the uterine serosa (IIIA), the T2W SI mass breaches the thin serosal surface. This can be difficult to detect if subtle, particularly if there are adjacent loops of bowel.

Disruption of the low T2W SI wall is suggestive of vaginal involvement (IIIB). In equivocal cases this is best evaluated at EUA.

Nodal disease.

Nodal spread is to the pelvic sidewall chains and para-aortic distribution (IIIC).

Stage IV disease: Bladder/rectal/distant metastases.

When the tumour invades the bladder, rectal mucosa or inguinal lymph nodes (IVA) or if there is distant metastatic disease (IVB).

4.4.2 Limitations/Pitfalls

- It can be difficult to comment on invasion in bulky tumours which distend the endometrium resulting in thinned, stretched myometrium, and if tumour extends into the cornua, the degree of invasion can be easily overestimated.
- Extensive leiomyomas (fibroids) can severely distort the endometrial cavity, making it difficult to see the disease and assess myometrial involvement accurately.
- Adenomyosis, a benign condition where the junctional zone is thickened and ill defined containing high T2W SI foci, can make extent of tumour involvement and depth of myometrial invasion difficult to determine.
- Sometimes it can be difficult to tell exactly where the cervix begins radiologically and therefore to know whether the cervix truly is involved if there is tumour in the region of the internal os.

4.4.2.1 CECT

Performed in patients with Type II histology and/or local imaging stage $\geq$ IB.

Metastatic disease is commonly peritoneal, and careful evaluation of the peritoneal surfaces and omentum is important. Evaluation of the chest is required to assess for metastatic disease particularly tumours of sarcomatous subtype.

4.4.3 Recurrent Disease

MRI is the best modality to establish whether there is tumour recurrence at the vaginal vault. The tumour will typically present as an intermediate soft tissue density mass. DWI is often very helpful in subtle cases. CECT is then performed to determine presence of metastatic disease. PET/CT is useful in equivocal cases or to determine suitability for salvage surgery or radiotherapy (Chap. 9).

4.5 Ovarian Cancer

4.5.1 Primary Diagnosis/Staging

Ovarian cancer is usually first detected as a complex mass on ultrasound. Suspicious features are of a cyst with septations, papillary projections or solid components which demonstrate vascularity. International ovarian tumour analysis (IOTA) simple rules may be used to identify US suspicious lesions [16].

A risk of malignancy index (RMI) may be used, combining US features with the Ca-125 and menopausal status [5]. If the RMI is high, i.e. appearances are

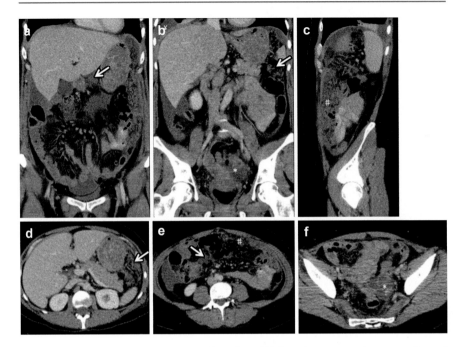

Fig. 4.4 37 year old female with stage IV disseminated high grade serous ovarian cancer. Coronal (**a, b**), sagittal (**c**) and axial (**d, e, f**) contrast-enhanced CT images demonstrating a solid-cystic left adnexal mass (*) with extensive omental (#) and peritoneal disease (*white arrows*). The *white arrow* in (**a**) demonstrates disease in the lesser sac while the arrow in (**d**) demonstrates deposits in the gastrosplenic ligament. Note is also made of ascites in the pelvis and right paracolic gutter and a right pleural effusion (¥). It was not possible to optimally debulk this patient at presentation and she was referred for chemotherapy

suspicious for malignancy, then staging is performed with CECT (Figs. 4.4 and 4.5), and patients are referred to the gynaecological oncology team for optimal treatment.

If the IOTA simple rules are not met or RMI is indeterminate, further characterisation with MRI may be helpful. Recommended sequences used to evaluate adnexal lesions are shown in Table 4.4 [15].

Adnexal mass characterisation is beyond the scope of this chapter; however, further details can be found in the literature [14]. Table 4.5 lists features of benign versus malignant disease. Figure 4.6 demonstrates several of the typical MRI features of a malignant ovarian lesion.

The preferred treatment for ovarian cancer is complete debulking surgery, with resection of all visible disease. If the disease is too extensive, then it is re-evaluated after chemotherapy to assess suitability for delayed debulking surgery.

The role of imaging in staging is to identify sites and extent of disease prior to surgery as this may help with surgical planning. If disease appears very advanced and is affecting sites which are less amenable to surgical resection (see Table 4.6), it is important to document as unsuccessful surgery delays the start of neoadjuvant chemotherapy.

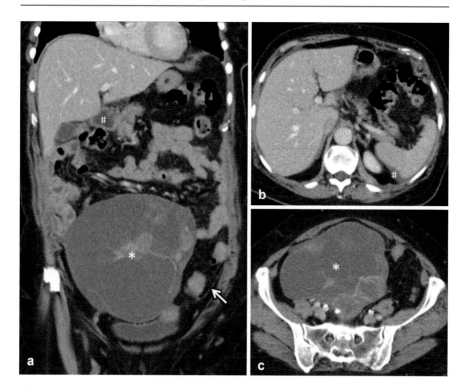

Fig. 4.5 40 year old female with stage IIIC high grade serous ovarian cancer. Coronal (**a**) and axial (**b**, **c**) contrast-enhanced CT images show a large complex predominantly cystic pelvic mass with numerous septations and solid internal components (*). There is streaky change noted in the peritoneal fat and omentum, small peritoneal nodules and fine enhancement of the peritoneal lining (*white arrow*, **a**). A small volume of ascites is also noted (#). In contrast to the patient shown in Figure 4.4 this lady had very little disease aside from the primary ovarian mass and was optimally debulked at initial surgery

Table 4.4 MRI sequences in adnexal mass characterisation

Sequence	Plane	Reason
T1W and T2W (renal hila to the symphysis pubis)	Axial (large FOV)	Evaluate para-aortic LN Assess for hydronephrosis Bone marrow (T1W)
T2W	Sagittal	Assess the uterus and fluid/peritoneal disease in pouch of Douglas
T2W	Axial oblique (small FOV, high resolution perpendicular to the uterus, known as ovarian axis)	Visualise both ovaries and assess the mass Nodal evaluation
T1W fat saturation	Axial	Assess for fat content
DWI	Axial	Look for areas of restriction in the mass and peritoneum
Dynamic contrast acquisition T1W fat saturation	Axial/sagittal	Assess for enhancement of solid components/septa

T1W T1-weighted, *T2W* T2-weighted, *DWI* diffusion-weighted imaging, *FOV* field of view, *LN* lymph node

Table 4.5 MRI characteristics of a malignant vs. benign ovarian mass

Malignant	Benign
Solid cystic mass	Cyst with no internal component
Measures >4 cm	Fat content (may indicate dermoid)
Wall thickness >3 mm	Low T2W SI walls/content (may suggest fibroma/cystadenofibroma)
Thickened enhancing septa	Low grade/no enhancement
Enhancing nodules/papillae	Layering (seen in haemorrhagic cysts/endometrioma)
Ancillary features: ascites, peritoneal disease and lymph nodes	

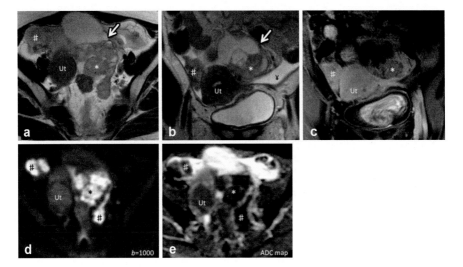

Fig. 4.6 55 year old female with disseminated ovarian cancer. Axial (**a**) and coronal (**b**) T2-weighted MR images show a solid-cystic left ovarian mass (*white arrow*). The solid components of the mass are of intermediate T2W signal intensity and show enhancement following gadolinium administration (*) on the coronal post-contrast T1-weighted fat suppressed image (**c**) and restriction (*) on the diffusion sequences (*b* = 1000 s/mm^2 (**d**) and corresponding apparent diffusion coefficient (ADC) map (**e**)). In addition, there are pelvic peritoneal tumour deposits (♯) which are of intermediate T2W signal, enhance following gadolinium and show restricted diffusion in line with the solid components of the primary tumour. Pelvic ascites is noted (¥). *Ut* Uterus

Table 4.6 Sites of peritoneal disease which may limit optimal debulking surgery

Subcapsular liver disease particularly subdiaphragmatic
Falciform ligament
Lesser sac
Gastrosplenic ligament
Small/large bowel mesentery
Small bowel serosal disease
Nodes above the renal hilum

The definition of which sites of disease are resectable varies between institutions and is dependent on local surgical expertise

If peritoneal disease is present, another important role of imaging is to identify a site for biopsy, most commonly this is the omentum.

Stage I disease: Tumour is confined to the adnexa.
A complex adnexal mass is present but with no evidence of peritoneal or nodal disease. Ascites may be present, and if positive on cytology, the tumour is grade IC.

Stage II disease: Tumour confined to the true pelvis.
There may be involvement of the fallopian tube, uterus and ascites. Pelvic peritoneal enhancement may be seen on CT, or thickening and discrete nodules may be present on MRI. DWI often demonstrates subtle disease well.

Stage III disease: Tumour elsewhere in the abdomen.
As the commonest route of metastatic spread is via the peritoneum, careful interrogation of the peritoneal surfaces is required, particularly the omentum, liver surface, gastrosplenic ligament, lesser sac and small and large bowel mesentery. Retroperitoneal nodal disease may be present (IIIA1).

Stage IV disease: Disease spreading beyond peritoneum and abdominal nodes.
Includes:

- Parenchymal liver metastases (as distinguished from subcapsular deposits); they should not contact the liver surface and are relatively uncommon in ovarian malignancy.
- Thoracic metastatic disease which includes cytologically positive pleural effusion and parenchymal pulmonary involvement.
- Involved paracardiac and inguinal lymph nodes.

4.5.2   Limitations/Pitfalls

- Diffuse small volume peritoneal disease (potentially inoperable) can be invisible/hard to appreciate. It is important to comment on peritoneal enhancement even if subtle.
- Careful evaluation of the gastrointestinal tract, pancreas and breasts is essential as primary tumours here can metastasise to the peritoneum and ovary. Correlation with a full panel of tumour markers is helpful.
- Benign entities that can mimic peritoneal disease include tuberculosis, dermoid rupture or oedematous omentum secondary to ascites.

4.5.3   Response Assessment

Follow-up is performed with CECT which can monitor peritoneal disease and demonstrate recurrent disease if suspected, e.g. if Ca-125 begins to rise, usually within the peritoneum.

4.6   Nodal Evaluation

Nodal evaluation with conventional CECT and MRI utilises size criteria with a short axis diameter of ≥10 mm considered pathological. These modalities have a high specificity (94 %) but a low sensitivity (40–60 %) as they fail to detect metastases in normal-sized nodes. Morphological features such as presence of necrosis, an irregular margin and nodal SI similar to the primary tumour can be used to evaluate smaller nodes, and knowledge of organ-specific nodal draining sites is important.

DWI is helpful in detecting lymph nodes, which are often restricted. Malignant involvement remains difficult to assess. In endometrial cancer, low ADC values within the lymph nodes similar to or less than that of the primary may infer tumour involvement, but sensitivity and specificity are unproven at present [11].

Key Points

Ultrasound (US) and magnetic resonance imaging (MRI) are the imaging modalities of choice for detailed investigation of the female pelvis.

Contrast-enhanced CT (CECT) plays an important role in the identification of disease beyond the uterus and ovaries, allowing evaluation of the peritoneal surfaces, omentum, upper abdominal viscera, thorax and nodal stations.

Cervical Cancer

Primary diagnosis/staging: MRI is the optimal imaging modality for pretreatment local staging of cervical cancer.

The most important sequences are high-resolution sagittal T2-weighted (T2W) series and an axial oblique sequence orientated perpendicular to the long axis of the cervix.

CECT of the chest, abdomen and pelvis is indicated in patients with advanced disease.

Follow-up: In patients treated with CRT, serial MRI can be used to monitor response.

Endometrial Cancer

Primary diagnosis/staging: Transvaginal ultrasound is the optimal method to demonstrate the endometrial cavity.

Once a histopathological diagnosis of malignancy has been established, local staging may be undertaken with MRI.

In patients with Type II histology and/or local imaging stage ≥ IB, contrast-enhanced CT is performed.

Limitations/pitfalls: Invasion in bulky tumours, extensive leiomyomas (fibroids) and adenomyosis.

Recurrent disease: MRI is the best modality to establish whether there is tumour recurrence at the vaginal vault.

PET/CT is useful in equivocal cases or to determine suitability for salvage surgery or radiotherapy.

Ovarian Cancer

Primary diagnosis/staging: Ultrasound is the first baseline test.

The role of imaging in staging is to identify sites and extent of disease prior to surgery as this may help with surgical planning.

Limitations/pitfalls: (a) diffuse small volume peritoneal disease and (b) benign entities that can mimic peritoneal disease.

Response assessment is performed with CECT which can monitor peritoneal disease and demonstrate recurrent disease if suspected.

References

1. Babar SA, et al. MRI appearances of recurrent cervical cancer. Eur Radiol. 2004;14:429.
2. Elit L, et al. Follow-up for women after treatment for cervical cancer. Curr Oncol. 2010;17(3):65–9.
3. Goldstein RB, et al. Evaluation of the woman with postmenopausal bleeding: society of radiologists in ultrasound-sponsored consensus conference statement. J Ultrasound Med. 2001; 20:1025–36.
4. Grigsby PW, Siegel BA, Dehdashti F. Lymph node staging by positron emission tomography in patients with carcinoma of the cervix. J Clin Oncol. 2001;19(17):3745–9.
5. Jacobs I, et al. A risk of malignancy incorporating CA 125, ultrasound and menopausal status for the accurate preoperative diagnosis of ovarian cancer. Br J Obstet Gynaecol. 1990;97(10):922–9.
6. Kaji Y, et al. Histopathology of uterine cervical carcinoma: diagnostic comparison of endorectal surface coil and standard body coil MRI. J Comput Assist Tomogr. 1994;18(5):785–92.
7. Kinkel K, et al. Radiologic staging in patients with endometrial cancer: a meta-analysis. Radiology. 1999;212(3):711–8.
8. Landoni F, et al. Randomised study of radical surgery versus radiotherapy for stage Ib-IIa cervical cancer. Lancet. 1997;350(9077):535–40.
9. London Cancer Alliance Guidelines. LCA Gynaecological Cancer Clinical Guidelines. 2014. Available at: http://www.londoncanceralliance.nhs.uk/media/75982/LCA_Gynaecology OncologyGuidelines2014.pdf (accessed September 2014.
10. Rechichi G, et al. Myometrial invasion in endometrial cancer: diagnostic performance of diffusion-weighted MR imaging at 1.5-T. Eur Radiol. 2010;20(3):754–62.
11. Rechichi G, et al. ADC maps in the prediction of pelvic lymph nodal metastatic regions in endometrial cancer. Eur Radiol. 2013;23(1):65–74.
12. Sala E, et al. Added value of dynamic contrast-enhanced magnetic resonance imaging in predicting advanced stage disease in patients with endometrial carcinoma. Int J Gynecol Cancer. 2009;19(1):141–6.
13. Scottish Intercollegiate Guidelines Network. Management of cervical cancer. (SIGN Guideline No 99). 2008. Available at: http://www.sign.ac.uk/guidelines/fulltext/99/index.html. Accessed Sept 2014.
14. Spencer J, et al. ESUR guidelines for MR imaging of the sonographically indeterminate adnexal mass: an algorithmic approach. Eur Radiol. 2009;20(1):25–35.
15. Thomassin-Naggara I, et al. Development and preliminary validation of an MRI scoring system for adnexal masses. Radiology. 2013;267(2):432–43.
16. Timmerman D, et al. Simple ultrasound rules to distinguish between benign and malignant ovarian masses before surgery: prospective validation by IOTA group. BMJ. 2010;341:c6839.

Basic Principles of PET-CT Imaging

5

Deborah Tout, John Dickson, and Andy Bradley

Contents

5.1   Introduction

PET-CT imaging has become a very powerful tool in cancer imaging, it utilises the detection of the radiation emitted from radionuclides that decay by positron (β^+) emission. This chapter looks into the physical principles of this technique, factors that affect the quality of the images produced and some of the artefacts and problems that may be encountered.

The original version of this chapter was revised: The erratum to this chapter is available at DOI 10.1007/978-3-319-29249-6_11

D. Tout (✉)
Biomedical Technology Services, Gold Coast University Hospital,
Southport, QLD, Australia
e-mail: Deborah.Tout@health.qld.gov.uk

J. Dickson
Department of Nuclear Medicine, University College London Hospitals
NHS Foundation Trust, London, UK

A. Bradley
Nuclear Medicine Centre, Manchester Royal Infirmary, Manchester, UK
e-mail: Andy.Bradley@cmft.nhs.uk

© Springer International Publishing Switzerland 2016
T. Barwick, A. Rockall (eds.), *PET/CT in Gynecological Cancers*,
Clinicians' Guides to Radionuclide Hybrid Imaging, DOI 10.1007/978-3-319-29249-6_5

5.2   Positron Emission Tomography (PET)

Positron emission tomography (PET) is the imaging of radiopharmaceuticals labelled with positron-emitting radionuclides. Positrons are the positively charged antimatter version of the electron and are ejected during the radioactive decay of a proton-rich nucleus; during this decay process, a proton in the nucleus is converted into a neutron. The positron is ejected from the nucleus carrying a lot of kinetic energy; it then travels a short distance and undergoes a number of interactions with the surrounding atoms. In each interaction, the positron loses some kinetic energy and changes its direction of travel, following a random path through the surrounding matter. When the positron is at rest, it annihilates with a nearby electron. Due to the conservation of energy, the energy associated with their combined mass (rest mass energy; $E = mc^2$) is converted to two annihilation photons each with energy of 511 keV. Conservation of momentum dictates that the two photons are emitted from the point of annihilation travelling in opposite directions (Fig. 5.1). These properties, the instantaneous production of two photons of equal energy travelling 180 degrees to each other, are the basis of the PET imaging technique used to localise where the original annihilation event occured within the patient.

A PET scanner is composed of several rings of small crystal scintillation detectors. Each detector is a few millimetres in size, and a group of them are formed into a block that is typically connected to a group of four photomultiplier tubes.

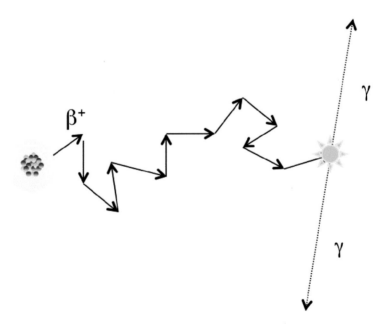

Fig. 5.1 During a nuclear decay, a positron is emitted from a nucleus and undergoes a series of interactions with atoms in the surrounding tissue. When its kinetic energy is almost zero, it and a neighbouring electron annihilate turning the mass of the two particles into energy in the form of two 511 keV photons. (Nucleus and random walk are not to scale)

The scintillator detectors convert incoming photons into light before amplifying the signal using the photomultiplier tubes. When there is a positron emission within the ring of detectors, the two 511 keV photons, travelling at the speed of light, will be detected almost instantaneously (within approximately 10 ns). Photons arriving at different detectors within this coincidence timing window are called coincidence events. The line between the two detectors that detected each coincidence event is called the 'line of response'. Typically data are collected over several minutes and all detected coincidence events are grouped into parallel lines of response to form projections through the patient that are used for image reconstruction, typically using iterative reconstruction techniques. The great advantage of this type of localisation is that, unlike a gamma camera, it does not require collimators to provide positional information and therefore offers much higher sensitivity than single-photon emission computed tomography (SPECT).

The type of coincidence event described above is called a 'true' coincidence, and it is these signals that create the useful image. There are, however, other unwanted coincidence events that can occur (Fig. 5.2). A 'random' coincidence event is where multiple positron emissions and annihilations occurring in quick succession lead to a number of photons arriving at the detectors within the coincidence time window. If the wrong pair of detected photons is seen as the coincidence event, this will lead to an incorrect line of response. This process is called a random event as the line of response is not associated with a true annihilation event. The proportion of random events to total coincidence events increases significantly with higher activity concentrations and larger coincidence acceptance time windows, e.g. by moving from 10 to 15 ns. A 'scattered' event is where one or both photons coming from a positron-electron annihilation are scattered during their path to the detectors; the line of response will again be incorrect. The fraction of coincidence events that can be attributed to scatter increases with increased scattering material i.e. larger or denser tissue. Although unwanted coincidences can degrade image quality, all modern image reconstruction techniques use correction algorithms, which limit the effect of these types of event.

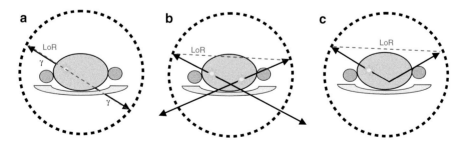

Fig. 5.2 Coincidence events in PET. (**a**) A true event with correct line of response (*LoR*), (**b**) a random event with two unrelated annihilations registering an incorrect line of response, (**c**) a scattered event where one photon has been scattered leading to an incorrectly positioned line of response

Along with adjustments for scattered and random events, there are other corrections that need to be applied during the reconstruction process to increase the accuracy of the final image. These include dead-time corrections to deal with the high count rates found in PET and a normalisation correction to correct for the difference in measured signal across pairs of detectors used to give the lines of response. However, the most dramatic of the corrections applied in PET is that to correct for photon attenuation within the patient. Although the photons in PET are more energetic than those in single-photon tomography, both photons need to be detected for a signal to be registered; this means that the full thickness of patient tissue traversed by both photons affects the relative attenuation of signal from different parts of the patient. The effects of photon attenuation are therefore more dramatic in PET than in SPECT and lead to the classic 'hot' skin and lungs on uncorrected images (Fig. 5.3).

Exact attenuation correction (AC) is relatively straightforward so long as an accurate attenuation map is known. With the advent of PET-CT, the CT scan, which effectively is a map of attenuation at x-ray energies, can, with appropriate conversion factors, provide attenuation correction maps in a matter of seconds. The CT is mounted in the same gantry as the PET, and the bed moves the patient between the two scanners for sequential imaging. There are issues to be considered when using attenuation maps derived from CT, such as accurate translation of attenuation coefficients from lower-energy x-ray photons to 511 keV; potential misregistration due to patient and respiratory motion; the use of contrast agents leading to incorrect attenuation maps owing to their enhanced attenuation only at the lower x-ray energies; and the presence of metal artefacts and the additional radiation dose to the patient. Despite these limitations, the use of CT for AC has grown rapidly because of the low statistical noise in the attenuation maps and the addition of registered anatomical information; the fusion of CT with PET greatly enhances the interpretation of the functional information as will be seen through most of this book.

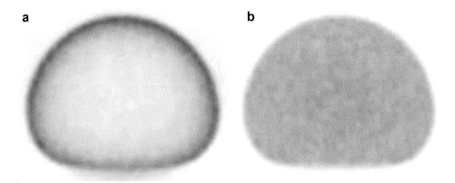

Fig. 5.3 Images of a transaxial slice through a phantom filled with a uniform solution of fluorine-18 (**a**) without correction for photon attenuation and (**b**) with attenuation correction

More recent technical advances include resolution (point-spread function) modelling in PET image reconstruction resulting in significant improvements in image resolution and contrast. Also modern fast crystal detectors are able to more precisely record the difference in the arrival times of the coincidence photons, known as time-of-flight (TOF) imaging. TOF helps localise the point of origin of the annihilation event along the line of response. The reduction in noise offered by TOF can be equated to a gain in sensitivity.

An advantage of applying a comprehensive set of corrections in PET-CT is that, with the inclusion of a sensitivity calibration, there is the possibility to calculate voxel values in terms of activity concentration per unit volume (kBq/ml). This activity concentration will change with patient size or administered activity so it becomes more useful if this uptake is represented as a value normalised by the available activity concentration in the body. This is achieved by normalising for injected activity and body size (weight or lean body mass), and this leads to the semi-quantitative index known as standardised uptake value (SUV). The SUV in each voxel will equal one for a uniform distribution. SUV is defined as

$$SUV(g/ml) = \frac{\text{activity concentration}(kBq/ml)}{\text{administered activity}(MBq)/\text{weight}(kg)}$$

SUV was defined for use in PET whole-body oncology imaging with fluorine-18-fluorodeoxyglucose (usually abbreviated as [^{18}F] FDG or just FDG). Most PET display workstations will display PET images in SUV. Although the use of SUV is widespread, there are many factors that can affect its accuracy. It requires accurate measurement of administered activity, injection time, scan time and patient weight and is affected by the performance characteristics of the PET scanner and image reconstruction factors. SUV also has a strong positive correlation with body weight. Heavy patients have a higher percentage of body fat that contributes to body weight but accumulates little FDG in the fasting state, so SUVs in non-fatty tissues are increased in larger patients. SUV normalised to lean body mass or body surface area has been shown to have a lesser dependence on body weight, although SUV normalised to body weight is still the most clinically used parameter. Many physiological factors can affect SUV, including scan delay time (accumulation of FDG continues to increase over time), patient's resting state, temperature, blood glucose level, insulin levels and renal clearance. In addition FDG is not a specific tumour marker, and uptake will be high in areas affected by infective or inflammatory processes that are often seen immediately post-chemotherapy.

Several values of SUV can be quoted, the most common being SUV_{max} which is robust and relatively independent of the observer, but as it refers to a single voxel value, it is strongly affected by image noise and can change significantly depending on count statistics and reconstruction parameters. It may also not be representative of the overall uptake in a heterogeneous tumour. SUV_{mean} is more representative of the average tumour uptake and is less affected by image noise, but can be prone to observer variability if freely drawn regions are used. Although the SUV formula has been criticised, the simplicity of the calculation makes it extremely attractive for routine clinical use.

There is a wide range of positron-emitting radionuclides used in PET (Table 5.1). Many have a short half-life, which requires an expensive cyclotron production facility on the same site as the PET-CT scanner. Fluorine-18 has a slightly longer half-life allowing it to be transported from the production facility to other imaging sites. This explains the popularity of fluorinated PET radiopharmaceuticals such as FDG. There are also longer half-life radionuclides such as copper-64 which allows imaging of pharmaceuticals with slower uptake kinetics. However, not all PET radionuclides require a cyclotron. Generators also exist, similar to the molybdenum-99/technetium-99 m generator, which can produce PET radionuclides repeatedly on site. Gallium-68 and rubidium-82 are popular, short-lived, generator-produced PET radionuclides; gallium-68 comes from germanium-68 parent and rubidium-82 from strontium-82 parent.

Not all radioactive decays result in the emission of a positron; for example, with copper-64, only 18 % of decays produce positrons. This means that the sensitivity of the PET scanner to copper-64-labelled compounds is less than a fifth of that possible with fluorine-18. There may also be additional radiations resulting from the other decay routes or contaminants which can affect patient and staff radiation exposure and image quality.

The average range of the positron is important as it determines the distance the positron travels before the creation of the annihilation photons; this range is dependent on the initial energy of the positron following the radioactive decay. Because the positron moves through the tissue in a random path, it is not possible to know the exact point in the tissue where the original decay took place. Spatial resolution in the images depends, to some extent, on the average range of the positron in that tissue. As a result, the spatial resolution of gallium-68 and rubidium-82 imaging will be worse than that from fluorine-18 tracers. The average positron ranges given in Table 5.1 are for soft tissue; the range of a positron will be much greater in air.

By far the most common radiopharmaceutical currently used in PET imaging is [F-18] FDG. Although FDG is a glucose analogue, it does not enter the glycolytic pathway after phosphorylation, but becomes trapped in the cell allowing imaging of FDG concentration, which infers glycolytic rate. Both glucose and FDG are filtered by the glomeruli, but unlike glucose, FDG is not reabsorbed by tubuli and therefore appears in urine. [F-18] FDG PET has become an important tool in oncology imaging for diagnosis, staging and to evaluate metabolic changes in tumours at the cellular level. Although very sensitive for imaging many cancer types, it is also non-specific, detecting many other physiological processes such as inflammation and infection.

Table 5.1 Properties of some radionuclides used in clinical PET imaging [1, 2]

Radionuclide	Half-life (min)	Average range (mm)	Positron fraction	Generator produced
Carbon-11	20.4	1.1	100	No
Nitrogen-13	9.96	1.5	100	No
Oxygen-15	2.03	2.5	100	No
Fluorine-18	110	0.6	97	No
Copper-64	762	0.6	18	No
Gallium-68	68	2.9	88	Yes
Rubidium-82	1.25	5.9	95	Yes

5.3   PET Scanning

PET-CT imaging usually starts with a localising scan projection radiograph often known as a 'scout' or 'topogram' where the extent of PET scanning is defined. The patient then has a CT scan of this defined length that will be used for attenuation correction and possibly uptake localisation, before moving through the scanner bore for the PET scan. The axial PET field of view which defines the amount of body that can be scanned in one stop is normally around 15 cm, although systems are now available that scan 22 cm or even 26 cm. For brain scanning or cardiac scanning, only one field of view is required; however in oncology imaging where the extent of disease is often of interest, whole-body imaging can be performed. This is typically done by acquiring several fields of view with a slight overlap to allow for the detector sensitivity losses at the edges of the field of view (Fig. 5.4). Each of these fields of view are called a bed position, and the time of each scan at these bed positions can be between 1.5 and 5 min in duration, depending on the affinity of the radiopharmaceutical and the sensitivity of the scanner. Patients should be made comfortable and immobilised when necessary to keep the patient in the same position to maintain registration between the PET and the CT used for attenuation correction and localisation and limit movement artefacts.

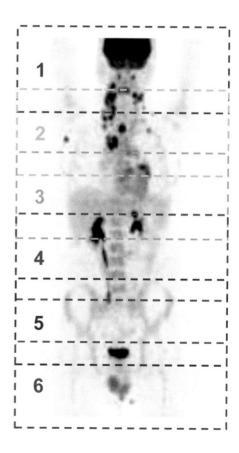

Fig. 5.4 A whole body image is made up of multiple bed positions that are stitched together; in this example six acquisitions are required to cover the desired length of the patient

For some applications, dynamic PET imaging over a single bed position can be useful to understand patient physiology. However, it is more typical to start PET imaging after a fixed period of time; this uptake or resting time is determined by the physiological uptake and excretion of the administered tracer with the aim to scan at the optimum time to have a good uptake in the target tissue with a low background circulation of the tracer in the rest of the body. For repeat imaging to assess disease progression, it is important to keep this uptake time duration similar for successive imaging, typically within +/− 5 min.

5.4   Imaging with [fluorine-18] FDG PET

The patient must arrive well hydrated and have fasted for between 4 and 6 h to ensure blood glucose levels are low prior to injection with FDG. This is to ensure that there is limited competition between FDG and existing blood glucose, so that uptake of FDG is maximised in order to give the best possible image quality. Care needs to be taken with diabetic patients. A patient history should be taken to determine when the patient last had radiotherapy or chemotherapy. FDG uptake can be elevated as a reactive response to these treatments. It is also important to remember that FDG can be sensitive to inflammation/infection, so a general understanding of the patients' wellbeing and history of recent physical trauma (including biopsy) is necessary. For SUV calculations, patients' weight (and height if correcting for lean body mass) should be taken with reliable calibrated instruments to ensure accurate quantification of uptake. Injection of FDG should be intravenous through an indwelling cannula and the clocks used to record the injection and scan times should be calibrated; any discrepancies in the recorded times can lead to errors in the decay correction used for quantification of the uptake. All PET tracers are beta emitters (a beta particle is a high energy electron or positron), so particular care should be taken to reduce the likelihood of extravasation and local radiation burden. To assist in the quantification of FDG uptake, the exact injected activity of FDG should be recorded.

Imaging typically starts at 60 min postinjection, and the patients must rest and be kept warm during this uptake period to avoid unwanted muscle or brown fat uptake. Patients are asked to void prior to imaging to reduce the activity in the bladder; full bladders containing high activity of FDG can cause difficulties in interpreting the images around this region and also increase the radiation dose to staff while the patient is positioned on the scanner bed. A multiple bed position whole-body scan is normally performed from mid-thigh up to the base of the brain. FDG is processed via renal excretion, so it is important where possible to scan in this direction to avoid scanning a bladder that has refilled with FDG during the scan. With the patient lying supine, whole-body imaging is performed with the arms raised above the patient's head to avoid CT beam-hardening artefacts and to ensure that the patient's body fits within the transaxial field of view. If head and neck imaging is required, an additional arms down scan over the head and neck area can be helpful to reduce attenuation in this area.

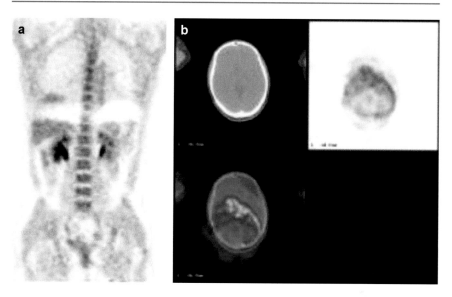

Fig. 5.5 (**a**) Respiratory motion artefact seen at the dome of the liver caused by mismatch of PET and CT for attenuation correction. (**b**) Patient motion between CT for attenuation correction and PET leading to poor correction for attenuation and localisation of tracer uptake

5.5   Artefacts

There are several artefacts that can occur in PET imaging even when all reasonable precautions are taken. One of the hardest artefacts to control is due to respiratory motion that can occur if the patient takes a large breath hold prior to or during the CT. As can be seen in Fig. 5.5a, the result can be a banana-shaped artefact caused by mismatch of PET and CT used for attenuation correction at the base of the lung and dome of the liver. The easiest way to avoid these artefacts is to ensure that the patient is relaxed prior to imaging and asking them not to take any large intakes of breath – particularly during the CT. Other motion-related artefacts are standard patient movement such as that seen in Fig. 5.5b. Relatively common in head and neck imaging, the mismatch of CT and PET can lead to incorrect attenuation correction and difficulty in localising features. Making the patient feel relaxed, helping them understand the need to remain still and appropriate immobilisation can help reduce the likelihood of these artefacts.

An artefact that cannot be easily controlled is the CT x-ray beam-hardening, and subsequent streaking aretefacts in the CT image, produced by metal prosthesis typically in the hip or where the patient has metal dental work (Fig. 5.6). Many modern systems have algorithms that can help minimise these effects. Nevertheless, care must be taken when quantifying uptake in affected areas because inaccuracies in the attenuation map derrived from the CT data can lead to inaccuracies in PET quantification. Another area where attenuation correction can fail is when CT contrast has been used. The conversion of the attenuation map derived from

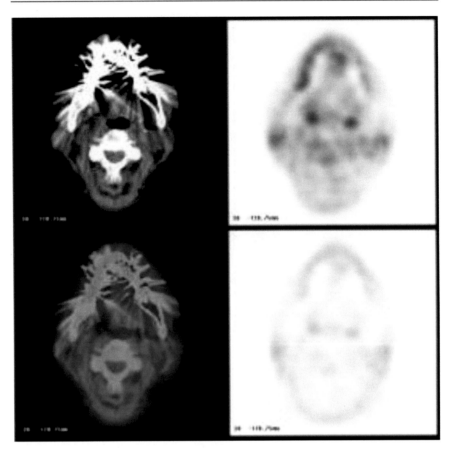

Fig. 5.6 Beam-hardening artefacts on CT caused by dental amalgam. PET quantification and localisation can be difficult although non-attenuation-corrected data (*bottom right panel*) may help with identifying artefacts in the attenuation-corrected images (*top right panel*)

CT x-ray energies to attenuation values at PET photon energies can fail in areas of CT contrast accumulation. This is due to the elevated attenuation of contrast media, such as iodine and barium, at the lower x-ray energies due to the k-edge absorption peak; this peak does not affect the absorption of the 511 keV PET photons. As the reconstruction algorithm cannot distinguish between the tissue that has a high density and less dense tissue containing CT contrast, the attenuation correction overcorrects areas containing contrast. This again can lead to errors in PET quantification. If quantification is particularly important, e.g. in a trial setting, the contrast CT should be performed last after the PET data is acquired, and the attenuation correction should be performed using a low-dose CT acquired before the contrast administration.

An important tool to identiy many artefacts introduced during the attenuation correction process is the reading of PET images without attenuation correction. Although these images are then not quantitative, they can be useful to highlight areas of artefact and to assess disease within the patient.

Careful consideration of radiation protection is important due to the high-energy annihilation photons. Over ten times the thickness of lead is required to shield PET photons compared to 140 keV photons, and, immediately post injection, the dose rate from a patient administered with fluorine-18 is ten times that of a patient administered with the same activity of technetium-99 m. Extremity dose to staff can be high when handling PET tracers due to the positron radiations.

The short physical half-lives of PET tracers result in a lower patient dose than might be expected. A typical administered activity of 350 MBq [F-18] FDG corresponds to an effective dose of approximately 7 mSv, and with ongoing improvements in PET detector technology and reconstruction methods, both imaging times and typical administered activities are decreasing. The required level of CT image quality (and therefore effective dose) depends on the use of the CT data. When the CT data are used solely for AC, patient doses can be extremely low (<1 mSv). A notable improvement in image quality (and dose increase) is required if the CT data are to be used for AC and anatomical localization (typically 3–8 mSv), and a further increase in both image quality and dose is required if the CT images are to be used for diagnostic purposes, usually with the addition of contrast agents (typically >15 mSv).

Key Points
- Positron emission tomography (PET) is the imaging of radiopharmaceuticals labelled with positron-emitting radionuclides.
- Positron decay leads to two 511 keV photons following annihilation of the emitted positron and a nearby electron.
- $E = mc^2$. Positron mass $= 9.109 \times 10^{-31}$ g, speed of light $= 2.9979 \times 10^8$ m/s, 1 eV $= 1.6 \times 10^{-19}$ J. You know you want to do the calculation.
- A PET scanner is composed of several rings of scintillation detectors.
- Coincident detection of the two photons in different detectors allows an image to be formed from information gleaned by tracking 'lines of response' between these detectors.
- TOF helps localise the point of origin of the annihilation event along the line of response. This helps to decrease noise, and thereby improve signal to noise ratio.
- The sensitivity of the scanner drops towards the edges of the axial field of view of the detectors. Adjacent bed positions need to be account to correct this.

- A semi-quantitative index, standardised uptake value (SUV) is commonly used in clinical PET.
- Several values of SUV can be quoted, the most common being SUV_{max} which is relatively robust, as it is less affected by the observer than SUV_{mean}, but it is strongly affected by image noise.
- SUV_{mean} is more representative of the average tumour uptake and is less affected by image noise but can be prone to observer variability.
- To assist in the quantification of FDG uptake, the exact injected activity of FDG should be recorded.
- For SUV calculations, patients' weight (and height if correcting by lean body mass) should be taken with reliable calibrated instruments to ensure accurate quantification of uptake.
- SUV values are affected by changes in reconstruction techniques and can vary between scanners; it is only semi-quantitative.
- Careful patient preparation is important to obtain good-quality PET images.
- All PET tracers are beta emitters, so particular care should be taken to reduce the likelihood of extravasation and local radiation burden.
- There are several artefacts that can occur in PET imaging; even when all reasonable precautions are taken, knowledge of these is important when interpreting images.
- The effects of photon attenuation are more dramatic in PET, and attenuation correction is essential.
- A typical administered activity of 350 MBq [F-18] FDG corresponds to an effective dose of approximately 7 mSv.
- Radiation doses to staff are much higher when exposed to PET tracers than from similar activities of other technetium-based nuclear medicine tracers.

References

1. NUDAT 2.6. National Nuclear Data Centre, Brookhaven National Laboratory. http://www.nndc.bnl.gov/nudat2/.
2. Cal-Gonzalez J, et al. Positron range effects in high resolution 3D PET imaging, Nuclear Science Symposium Conference Record (NSS/MIC). 2009 IEEE. Orlando, FL.

^{18}F-FDG and Non-FDG PET Radiopharmaceuticals

6

James Ballinger and Gopinath Gnanasegaran

Contents

6.1   Introduction

Positron emission tomography/computed tomography (PET/CT) is one of the key imaging techniques in oncology. Hybrid PET/CT provides both structural and metabolic information and in general improves sensitivity, specificity and reporter confidence.

Fluorine-18 (^{18}F) is the most commonly used PET-emitting radionuclide label in clinical practice. It is produced using a cyclotron and has a physical half-life of 110 min. The most widely used tracer at present is the glucose analogue, 2-fluoro-2-deoxyglucose (FDG) (Table 6.1).

The original version of this chapter was revised: The erratum to this chapter is available at DOI 10.1007/978-3-319-29249-6_11

J. Ballinger (✉)
Division of Imaging Sciences, King's College London, London, UK
e-mail: Jim.ballinger@kcl.ac.uk

G. Gnanasegaran
Department of Nuclear Medicine, Royal Free London NHS Foundation Trust, London, UK

© Springer International Publishing Switzerland 2016
T. Barwick, A. Rockall (eds.), *PET/CT in Gynecological Cancers*,
Clinicians' Guides to Radionuclide Hybrid Imaging, DOI 10.1007/978-3-319-29249-6_6

Table 6.1 Oncology PET Radiopharmaceuticals [1–11]

Class	Radiopharmaceutical	Clinical application
Oncology: [18]F		
	Fludeoxyglucose (FDG)	Glucose metabolism
	Fluoride	Bone metabolism
	Fluoro-L-thymidine (FLT)	DNA synthesis
	Fluoromethylcholine (FCh)	Phospholipid synthesis
	Fluoroethylcholine (FEC)	Phospholipid synthesis
	Fluoroethyltyrosine (FET)	Protein synthesis
	Fluoromisonidazole (FMISO)	Hypoxia
	Fluoroazomycin arabinoside (FAZA)	Hypoxia
	Fluoroerythronitroimidazole (FETNIM)	Hypoxia
	Fluciclatide	Angiogenesis
	F-galacto-RGD	Angiogenesis
	Fluciclovine (FACBC)	Amino acid transport
	ICMT11	Apoptosis
Oncology: [11]C		
	Acetate	Membrane synthesis
	Choline	Phospholipid synthesis
	Methionine	Protein synthesis
Oncology: [68]Ga		
	DOTATOC	Somatostatin receptor
	DOTATATE	Somatostatin receptor
	HA-DOTATATE	Somatostatin receptor
	DOTANOC	Somatostatin receptor
	SOMATOSCAN	Somatostatin receptor
	PSMA	Prostate-specific membrane antigen
	NOTA-RGD	Angiogenesis
Oncology: [124]I		
	Iodide	Sodium-iodide symporter
	MIBG	Neuronal activity

6.2 PET Radiopharmaceuticals

6.2.1 ^{18}F-FDG

^{18}F-FDG has a role in localising, characterising, staging, monitoring treatment response and evaluation of recurrent disease in a variety of cancer types. However, increased FDG uptake is not specific to cancer cells. FDG accumulates in cells, in proportion to glucose utilisation [1–5]. In general, increased glucose uptake is a characteristic of most cancers and is in part mediated by overexpression of the GLUT-1 glucose transporter and increased hexokinase activity [1–5]. The net result is an increased accumulation of FDG within tumour cells at a rate greater than in normal tissue. Active inflammatory changes can also result in increased FDG uptake, due to increased glucose utilisation by activated granulocytes and mono-nuclear cells [1–5] (Tables 6.1, 6.2 and 6.3). The principal route of excretion of

Table 6.2 Properties of positron-emitting radionuclides used in clinical practice

Radionuclide	Half-life	Positron energy (max, MeV)	Other emissions	Means of production
Carbon-11	20 min	0.96	–	Cyclotron
Nitrogen-13	10 min	1.20	–	Cyclotron
Oxygen-15	2 min	1.74	–	Cyclotron
Fluorine-18	110 min	0.63	–	Cyclotron
Copper-62	10 min	2.93	–	Generator
Copper-64	13 h	0.65	Beta, gamma	Cyclotron
Gallium-68	68 min	1.83	–	Generator
Rubidium-82	76 s	3.15	–	Generator
Zirconium-89	79 h	0.40	Gamma	Cyclotron
Iodine-124	4.2 days	1.50	Gamma	Cyclotron

Table 6.3 Common radiopharmaceuticals and their mechanism of uptake [11]

Radiotracer	Mechanism of uptake
^{18}F-fluorodeoxyglucose (FDG)	Uptake by GLUT-1 transporter followed by phosphorylation by hexokinase
Sodium ^{18}F-fluoride (NaF)	Incorporated within hydroxyapatite in proportion to bone metabolism
^{68}Ga-labelled peptides	Bind to peptide receptor, most commonly somatostatin receptor
^{18}F-choline (FCh) ^{11}C-choline	Incorporation into phosphatidyl choline as part of cell wall synthesis
^{11}C-methionine	Amino acid transport
^{18}F-fluorothymidine (FLT) ^{11}C-thymidine	Phosphorylated by thymidine kinase in proliferating cells; FLT not incorporated into DNA
^{82}Rb-chloride	Transported into myocardial cells by sodium-potassium ATPase in proportion to regional myocardial perfusion

FDG from the bloodstream is via the urinary tract. The biodistribution of ^{18}F-FDG varies on several factors such as (a) fasting state, (b) medications, (c) duration of the uptake period post-tracer injection, (d) variant metabolism and (e) incidental pathology and is discussed in detail in Chap. 8.

6.3   Non-FDG Radiopharmaceuticals

In addition to ^{18}F-FDG, there are several cyclotron and generator-based radiolabelled molecules used in clinical PET/CT imaging. Sodium fluoride (^{18}F-NaF), ^{68}Ga-labelled peptides, ^{18}F-choline, ^{11}C-choline, etc., each have clinical applications and are discussed in detail in this pocketbook series titled *PET Radiotracers*. While FDG is the workhorse of oncological PET imaging, it is nonspecific as it monitors the ubiquitous process of glucose metabolism. Alternative tracers tend to be more specific in their targeting and application. Some attempt to probe the hallmarks of cancer, such as uncontrolled proliferation, angiogenesis, evasion of apoptosis and tissue invasion.

Tumour microenvironment, such as hypoxia, has also been probed. However, the tracers which have come into wider use tend to be those which monitor specific features such as membrane synthesis incorporating choline, prostate-specific membrane antigen (PSMA) expression and somatostatin receptor expression.

Conclusion

It is likely that the range of positron-emitting radiopharmaceuticals in routine clinical use will continue to expand in the coming years.

Key Points

- Fluorine-18 (^{18}F) is the most commonly used PET-emitting radionuclide label in clinical practice.
- Fluorine-18 (^{18}F) is produced using a cyclotron and has a physical half-life of 110 min.
- Most widely used tracer at present is the glucose analogue, 2-fluoro-2-deoxyglucose (FDG). FDG is the workhorse of oncological PET imaging.
- FDG is actively transported into the cell mediated by a group of structurally related glucose transport proteins (GLUT).
- Increased FDG uptake is not specific to cancer cells and often will accumulate in areas with increased metabolism and glycolysis.
- The principal route of excretion of FDG from the bloodstream is via the urinary tract.
- Non-FDG tracers include sodium fluoride (^{18}F-NaF), ^{68}Ga-labelled peptides, ^{18}F-choline, and ^{11}C-choline.

References

1. Torizuka T, Tamaki N, Inokuma T, et al. In vivo assessment of glucose metabolism in hepatocellular carcinoma with FDG-PET. J Nucl Med. 1995;36:1811–7.
2. Cook GJ, Fogelman I, Maisey MN. Normal physiological and benign pathological variants of ^{18}F-FDG PET scanning: potential for error in interpretation. Semin Nucl Med. 1996;26:308–14.
3. Warburg O. On the origin of cancer cells. Science. 1956;123:309–14.
4. Cook GJ, Maisey MN, Fogelman I. Normal variants, artefacts and interpretative pitfalls in PET imaging with ^{18}F-fluoro-2-deoxyglucose and carbon-11 methionine. Eur J Nucl Med. 1999;26:1363–78.
5. Culverwell AD, Scarsbrook AF, Chowdhury FU. False-positive uptake on 2-[^{18}F]-fluoro-2-deoxy-D-glucose (FDG) positron-emission tomography/computed tomography (PET/CT) in oncological imaging. Clin Radiol. 2011;66:366–82.
6. Shreve PD, Anzai Y, Wahl RL. Pitfalls in oncologic diagnosis with FDG PET imaging: physiologic and benign variants. Radiographics. 1999;19:61–77.
7. Delbeke D, Coleman RE, Guiberteau MJ, et al. Procedure guideline for tumour Imaging with ^{18}F-FDG PET/CT 1.0. J Nucl Med. 2006;47:885–95.

8. Boellaard R, O'Doherty MJ, Weber WA, et al. FDG PET and PET/CT: EANM procedure guidelines for tumour PET imaging: version 1.0. Eur J Nucl Med Mol Imaging. 2010; 37:181–200.
9. Segall G, Delbeke D, Stabin MG, et al. SNM practice guideline for sodium ^{18}F-fluoride PET/CT bone scans 1.0. J Nucl Med. 2010;51:1813–20.
10. Virgolini I, Ambrosini V, Bomanji JB, et al. Procedure guidelines for PET/CT tumour imaging with ^{68}Ga-DOTA-conjugated peptides: ^{68}Ga-DOTA-TOC, ^{68}Ga-DOTA-NOC, ^{68}Ga-DOTA-TATE. Eur J Nucl Med Mol Imaging. 2010;37:2004–10.
11. Juweid ME, Cheson BD. Positron-emission tomography and assessment of cancer therapy. N Engl J Med. 2006;2(354):496–507.

PET/CT Imaging: Patient Instructions and Preparation

7

Shaunak Navalkissoor, Thomas Wagner,
Gopinath Gnanasegaran, Teresa A. Szyszko,
and Jamshed Bomanji

Contents

7.1   Introduction

^{18}F-FDG PET is a frequently used imaging modality in the evaluation of cancer patients. A high-quality study performed ^{18}F-FDG PET study should be repeatable (same result produced if imaged on the same system) and reproducible (similar result if imaged at different sites). An essential component of this is adequate patient preparation to ensure study reproducibility and technical quality. Rigorous instructions

The original version of this chapter was revised: The erratum to this chapter is available at DOI 10.1007/978-3-319-29249-6_11

S. Navalkissoor (✉) • T. Wagner • G. Gnanasegaran
Department of Nuclear Medicine, Royal Free London NHS Foundation Trust, London, UK
e-mail: s.navalkissoor@nhs.net

T.A. Szyszko
Division of Imaging Sciences and Biomedical Engineering,
Nuclear Medicine and Radiology Clinical PET Centre, St Thomas' Hospital,
Kings College London, London, UK

J. Bomanji
Department of Nuclear Medicine, University College London Hospitals NHS Foundation Trust, London, UK

© Springer International Publishing Switzerland 2016
T. Barwick, A. Rockall (eds.), *PET/CT in Gynecological Cancers*,
Clinicians' Guides to Radionuclide Hybrid Imaging, DOI 10.1007/978-3-319-29249-6_7

63

Table 7.1 Contents of PET/CT request [1–5]

1. Patient name, date of birth, address and hospital identifier number
2. Clinical indication
3. Clinical question to be answered
4. Oncological history: site of tumour (if known), recent biopsy (site, date of biopsy and results if known, etc.), co-morbidity
5. Drug allergies, allergy to contrast agents
6. Diabetes status, if relevant (IDDM, NIDDM), and treatment
7. Renal function
8. Therapeutic interventions: type and date of last treatment (chemotherapy, surgery, radiotherapy, bone marrow stimulants and steroid administration)
9. Result and availability of previous imaging
10. Height and body weight
11. Referring clinician's contact details: (a) to discuss about the referral, (b) to contact during emergency and (c) to send the reports
12. Date at which results of the PET or PET/CT study must be available

should be followed regarding patient procedure. In addition, adequate referral information is important so that the correct timing of study and imaging protocol can be followed, e.g. lung gating for a base of lung lesion. This section addresses some of these issues, and summaries of required clinical information, patient preparation, procedure and imaging parameters are shown in Tables 7.1, 7.2 and 7.3.

FDG is a glucose analogue and is transferred intracellularly by glucose transporters. Many tumour cells overexpress glucose transporter proteins and hexokinase intracellularly, which allows FDG to be used to image these tumours.

7.2   Patient Preparation

One of the main aims in patient preparation is to reduce the hyperinsulinemic state, which occurs with recent glucose ingestion. Increased glucose levels cause competitive inhibition of ^{18}F-FDG uptake by the cells leading to decreased tumour (or other active process) to background ratio. Also increased insulin secondary to elevated blood glucose increases translocation of GLUT4, thereby shunting ^{18}F-FDG to organs with high density of insulin receptors (e.g. skeletal muscles). Patients should thus fast for at least 6 h prior to the study to ensure low insulin levels. Recent EANM guidelines suggest that patients with blood glucose <11 mmol/L can have FDG administered, whilst patients with glucose >11 mmol/L need to be rescheduled. Patients with diabetes (particularly with insulin-based treatments) need to be carefully scheduled to avoid a hyperinsulinemic state. (An example of scheduling includes a late morning appointment with an early breakfast and insulin injection.)

If glucose control is not achieved, then the PET scan can be rescheduled.

Another patient preparation also aims to reduce tracer uptake in normal tissues, thus increasing target-nontarget uptake. Patients should be hydrated adequately to decrease the concentration of FDG in the urine, decreasing artefacts and potentially reducing radiation dose. Drinking water is permitted; however, flavoured water contains sugar and cannot be consumed prior to the PET scan. Patients should be advised to dress warmly on the way to the PET suite and should be kept in a warm

Table 7.2 General instructions for an ^{18}F-FDG PET scan [1–5]

Appointment:
1. Send leaflets related to the scan and instructions
2. Confirm appointment
3. Medications list if any
4. History of diabetes, fasting state, recent infection/intervention, etc.

Before arrival:
1. Fast, except for water (for at least 6 h before the injection of ^{18}F-FDG and for most studies, at least 4 h before dedicated neuroimaging), avoid chewing gum
   (a) Morning appointment: patient should not eat after midnight [preferably have a light meal (no alcohol) during the evening prior to the PET study]
   (b) Afternoon appointment PET study: patient may have a light breakfast before 8.00 a.m. (no sugars or sugar-containing fillings/products)
2. Advise adequate pre-hydration
3. Intravenous fluids containing dextrose or parenteral feedings should be withheld for 4–6 h before radiotracer injection
4. Consider if intravenous contrast material is to be used for CT

Before injecting:
1. The blood glucose level should be checked and documented
   FDG PET study can be performed: if plasma glucose level is <11 mmol/L (or <200 mg/dL)
   FDG PET study should be rescheduled: if plasma glucose level is ≥11 mmol/L (or >200 mg/ dL) depending on patient's circumstances
2. Keep the patient in a warm room for 30–60 min before the injection and during the uptake period and maintain warmth with blankets during scan to reduce uptake in the brown fat. *(Lorazepam, diazepam and beta-blockers may help to reduce uptake by brown fat uptake if problematic)*
3. Check patient's ability to lie still for the duration of the scan and ability to put his or her arms overhead
4. Ask for history of claustrophobia
5. If intravenous contrast material is to be used, patients should be screened for iodinated contrast material allergy, renal disease and use of metformin for diabetes mellitus treatment
6. Take a brief history and document site of malignancy, including recent investigations and treatment history: surgery, radiation and chemotherapy

Table 7.3 ^{18}F-FDG PET/CT imaging parameters [1–5]

Routine imaging: skull base to upper thigh

Additional views: lower limbs views, dedicated head and neck or occasionally scan to the vertex is acquired as necessary

Brain imaging is frequently omitted in many institutions routinely (poor sensitivity of FDG PET for brain metastases)

Typical adult-administered activities: 185–370 MBq (5–10 mCi), up to 400 MBq

Largest effective dose administered: urinary bladder

Whole body effective dose of PET study is approximately 0.02 mSv/MBq or 7–8 mSv for an adult-administered activity of 370 MBq. CT dose depends on local protocol

room prior to the administration of FDG. This is to avoid accumulation of FDG in activated brown fat. In some cases with no contraindications to oral beta-blockers, propranolol (1 mg/kg, maximum 40 mg) should be given at least 90 min before FDG injection to reduce FDG uptake in brown adipose tissue. This is especially important in young patients. Strenuous physical activity should be avoided for at

Table 7.4 Example of low-carbohydrate, high-fat diet provided to patients prior to FDG PET cardiac imaging

Do not eat the following:

Sugar in any form (including natural sugars in fruits)

No starches, e.g. pasta, breads, cereals, rice and potatoes

No vegetables with high-carbohydrate content, no carrots or beetroot

No chocolates, sweets, chewing gums, mints and cough syrups

No processed products, e.g. processed deli meats

No sweetener substitutes like canderel or splenda

No milk or milk products

No cheese or cheese products

No nuts

No fruits

No alcohol

You can eat the following:

Poultry: fatty unsweetened chicken and turkey (fried or boiled, NOT grilled)

Meats: fatty unsweetened red meat, bacon, ham (fried or boiled, NOT grilled)

Fish: any fish (fatty unsweetened, fried or boiled, NOT grilled)

Shellfish: any non-processed shellfish

Eggs: fried, scrambled preparation without milk, omelette prepared without milk or vegetables

Butter and margarine

Vegetables: cucumber, broccoli, lettuce, celery, mushroom, green pepper, cabbage, spinach, asparagus, radish

Drinks: mineral water (still or sparkling), coffee, tea, herbal tea (without milk or sugar)

least 6 h prior to the scan to avoid excessive skeletal uptake. During the uptake period, the patient should not talk and avoid reading or chewing, to minimise uptake in these respective muscles.

If a lesion near the myocardium or the myocardium itself is being evaluated for suspected disease, careful patient preparation is required to limit cardiac uptake. A low-carbohydrate, high-fat, high-protein diet for at least 24 h before the scan (Table 7.4) and extended fasting for 18 h before the scan are recommended to switch the myocardial energy substrate from glucose to fatty acids. This is coupled with one or two intravenous bolus of heparin (50 IU/kg) given 90 min prior to ^{18}F-FDG injection for suppression of myocardial FDG uptake.

Review of patient's medication should be performed, e.g. steroids in high doses may cause hyperglycaemic states and in patients with suspected vasculitis may reduce the sensitivity of the test; metformin may cause diffuse large bowel uptake due to increased glucose utilisation of the intestinal mucosa. If intravenous contrast is going to be administered, metformin needs to be withheld on the day of the test and for a further 48 h.

7.3   Timing of FDG PET Scan After Treatment

When the PET scan is being protocolled, adequate information about previous treatments should be available to the authoriser to ensure accurate timing, e.g. in chemotherapy response assessments in lymphoma, the FDG PET scan should not be performed too early to avoid false negatives due to tumour stunning or false positives due to inflammatory uptake. An interval of at least 10 days should be allowed post-chemotherapy (interim PET) or at least 3 weeks at the end of chemotherapy to allow evaluation of response to chemotherapy. If patients are undergoing radiotherapy, the recommended post-therapy interval is 2–3 months.

Key Points
- Rigorous instructions should be followed regarding patient procedure.
- Adequate referral information is important so that the correct timing of study and imaging protocol can be followed.
- Increased glucose levels cause competitive inhibition of ^{18}F-FDG uptake.
- Increased insulin secondary to elevated blood glucose increases translocation of GLUT4.
- Patients should thus fast for at least 6 h prior to the study to ensure low insulin levels.
- Patients with blood glucose <11 mmol/L can have FDG administered, whilst patients with glucose >11 mmol/L need to be rescheduled (EANM guidelines).
- Patients with diabetes (particularly with insulin-based treatments) need to be carefully scheduled to avoid a hyperinsulinemic state.
- Patients should be hydrated adequately to decrease the concentration of FDG in the urine, decreasing artefacts and potentially reducing radiation dose.
- Keep the patient in a warm room for 30–60 min before the FDG injection.
- Strenuous physical activity should be avoided for at least 6 h prior to the scan.
- An interval of at least 10 days should be allowed post-chemotherapy (interim PET) or at least 3 weeks at the end of chemotherapy to allow evaluation of response to chemotherapy.
- In patients undergoing radiotherapy, the recommended post-therapy interval is 2–3 months.

References

1. Delbeke D, Coleman RE, Guiberteau MJ, et al. Procedure guideline for tumour imaging with ^{18}F-FDG PET/CT 1.0. J Nucl Med. 2006;47(5):885–95.
2. Boellaard R, O'Doherty MJ, Weber WA, et al. FDG PET and PET/CT: EANM procedure guidelines for tumour PET imaging: version 1.0. Eur J Nucl Med Mol Imaging. 2010;37(1): 181–200.
3. Boellaard R, Delgado-Bolton R, Oyen WGJ, Giammarile F, Tatsch K, Eschner W, et al. FDG PET/CT: EANM procedure guidelines for tumour imaging: version 2.0. Eur J Nucl Med Mol Imaging. 2015;42:328–54.

4. Juweid ME, Cheson BD. Positron-emission tomography and assessment of cancer therapy. N Engl J Med. 2006;354(5):496–507.
5. Graham MM, Wahl RL, Hoffmans JM, Yaps JT, Sunderland JT, et al. Summary of the UPICT protocol for ^{18}F-FDG PET/CT imaging in oncology clinical trials. J Nucl Med. 2015; 56:955–61.

¹⁸F-FDG PET/CT Imaging: Normal Variants, Pitfalls and Artefacts

8

Kanhaiyalal Agrawal, Gopinath Gnanasegaran, Evangelia Skoura, Alexis Corrigan, and Teresa A. Szyszko

Contents

8.1   Introduction

In recent years, positron emission tomography (PET)/computed tomography (CT) has gained widespread clinical acceptance in oncology. It is being used extensively in the diagnosis, staging, restaging and therapy response evaluation of tumours (Table 8.1) along with several benign indications in cardiology and neurology.

The original version of this chapter was revised: The erratum to this chapter is available at DOI 10.1007/978-3-319-29249-6_11

K. Agrawal (✉)
Department of Nuclear Medicine and PET/CT, North City Hospital, Kolkata, India
e-mail: drkanis@gmail.com

G. Gnanasegaran
Department of Nuclear Medicine, Royal Free London NHS Foundation Trust, London, UK

E. Skoura
Department of Nuclear Medicine, Institute of Nuclear Medicine, UCLH, London, UK

A. Corrigan
Department of Nuclear Medicine and Radiology, Maidstone and Tunbridge Wells NHS Trust, Tunbridge Wells, UK

T.A. Szyszko
Division of Imaging Sciences and Biomedical Engineering, Nuclear Medicine and Radiology, Clinical PET Centre, St Thomas' Hospital, Kings College London, London, UK

© Springer International Publishing Switzerland 2016
T. Barwick, A. Rockall (eds.), *PET/CT in Gynecological Cancers*,
Clinicians' Guides to Radionuclide Hybrid Imaging, DOI 10.1007/978-3-319-29249-6_8

69

Table 8.1 Clinical role of PET/CT imaging in oncology

Diagnosis
Localisation
Staging
Restaging
Treatment response
Recurrent disease or relapse
Radiotherapy planning
Guiding metabolic biopsy
Grading tumours

Fluorine-18 (^{18}F) 2-fluoro-2-deoxy-D-glucose (FDG) is the most commonly used positron-emitting radiotracer in PET/CT studies. In this chapter, we will mainly focus on normal variants and artefacts in ^{18}F-FDG PET/CT studies.

^{18}F-FDG is a glucose analogue labelled with a positron-emitting isotope ^{18}F. It is transported into cells through glucose transporters and phosphorylated by enzyme hexokinase to ^{18}F-FDG-6-phosphate [1]. The cell membrane is impermeable to both glucose-6-phosphate and ^{18}F-FDG-6-phosphate. However, the latter cannot be degraded further via the glycolysis pathway and remains trapped within the cell. ^{18}F-FDG is accumulated in malignant tissues more avidly than within the normal tissues due to increased glucose metabolism rate, increased expression of glucose transporters and highly active hexokinase bound to the mitochondria of the malignant tissue in comparison to the normal tissue. However, ^{18}F-FDG uptake is also known to occur in inflammation, infection and healing tissues. This is partly due to the fact that infiltrated granulocytes and tissue macrophages use glucose as energy source. In inflammation, the granulocytes and macrophages are activated, and hence, glucose metabolism increases [2].

There can be variable degree of physiological tracer uptake in the various organs in the ^{18}F-FDG PET/CT scans (Fig. 8.1, Tables 8.2, 8.3, 8.4, and 8.5) [3–16]. Recognition of physiological tracer distribution is essential in avoiding incorrect image interpretation. Sometimes special patient preparation is needed to suppress the physiological tracer uptake to identify pathology in some organs [14]. It is important that patient is relaxed on the day of the study and should maintain silence to avoid muscle uptake [5]. Brown fat uptake can be suppressed by keeping the patient warm or sometimes by administration of oral beta-blockers and benzodiazepines, especially in patients with suspected pathology in the neck and mediastinum. Similarly, cardiac ^{18}F-FDG PET imaging needs either prolonged fasting or special low-carbohydrate high-fat diet to suppress physiological uptake in the myocardium [14]. It is always better to avoid administering insulin to the patient on the day of study as this may lead to increased background activity in the fat and muscles and decreases uptake in the tumour [5]. Physiological tracer activity in the urinary tract may mask pathological conditions. Good hydration and the use of intravenous diuretics should be considered to decrease the urinary stasis in the kidneys and ureters. It also dilutes the urine activity in the urinary bladder and helps in better evaluation of surrounding structures like the prostate gland.

^{18}F-FDG PET study immediately after chemotherapy and radiotherapy introduces false-positives findings [5–9, 12, 13, 16]. Hence, at least a gap of 3 weeks following chemotherapy and 3 months following radiotherapy to perform ^{18}F-FDG

Table 8.2 ¹⁸F-FDG PET scan appearances and physiological variation [5–9, 12, 13, 16]

Organ	Physiological uptake/variation	Comments
Brain	Intense uptake in the cortex, basal ganglia and thalami (Figs. 8.1 and 8.2a)	Metastases are best assessed with MRI
Breast	Low-grade diffuse uptake within the breast is normal due to proliferative glandular tissue. Higher uptake may be seen in adolescent girls with dense breasts (Fig. 8.2d) The uptake in the areola is variable, but prominent uptake may be seen	Markedly increased in lactating breast. The amount of radioactivity within milk from the breasts is low. The infant is more likely to receive radiation exposure from close contact with the breast, rather than from milk
Bone marrow	Low-diffuse uptake in haematopoietic bone marrow is physiological	
Brown fat	Neck, paraspinal, retroperitoneal fat, etc.	Patient waiting areas should be kept warm. Drug intervention may be helpful
Endometrium	Central moderate uptake within the uterus is normal during ovulatory and secretory phases	Menstrual history is important and tracer uptake may be pathological in postmenopausal women
GI tract	Highly variable Increased tracer uptake with a focal, diffuse, or segmental distribution could be physiological and more marked in patients taking the antidiabetic drug such as metformin (Fig. 8.15)	Focal areas of increased uptake usually warrant further evaluation
Heart	Variable ranging from negligible to intense uptake (Fig. 8.3) depending on its metabolic state at the time of the study	Partly depends on fasting state (may be suppressed by prolonged fast or low-carbohydrate high-fat diet). However, in PET cardiac imaging, the main aim is to increase cardiac uptake of FDG, and increasing uptake in cardiac cells can be achieved by increasing the serum insulin level or decreasing the free fatty acid level
Liver	Mild-to-moderate uptake (relatively homogeneous) (Fig. 8.2e)	
Muscles	Mild uptake is physiological Symmetrical diaphragmatic, intercostal and strap muscle uptake could be physiological or may relate to increased respiratory effort in patients with pulmonary disease (Fig. 8.4)	Tracer uptake is increased in patients who are not adequately fasted or following exercise/exertion (thorough clinical history is useful in these cases) (Fig. 8.5)
Ovary	During the midcycle, moderate increased uptake in the adnexae is normal (unilateral or bilateral) (Fig. 8.6)	Menstrual history is important. Tracer uptake may be pathological in postmenopausal women. Bilateral adnexal and uterine activity is likely to represent physiological ovarian and uterine uptake in a premenopausal woman
Ocular muscles	Moderate or intense tracer uptake Related to eye movement during uptake period (Fig. 8.2b)	Patient should be advised to rest quietly in darkened room

(continued)

Table 8.2 (continued)

Organ	Physiological uptake/variation	Comments
Salivary glands	Low-grade tracer uptake is physiological and is often symmetrical	
Spleen	Homogeneous uptake slightly less than the liver (Fig. 8.2e)	
Testes	Mild-to-moderate symmetrical uptake is physiological and declines with age (Fig. 8.2h)	
Thymus	Low-to-moderate uptake in children and young adults is normal (Fig. 8.7)	Often reactivated post-chemotherapy and tracer uptake should be correlated with age of the patient and medical history/treatment
Thyroid	Diffuse or focal uptake is often seen (Fig. 8.11d)	Diffuse uptake is seen in patients with Graves' disease, subacute thyroiditis or Hashimoto's thyroiditis. Focal uptake is often seen in thyroid nodules and should be further evaluated with fine needle aspiration to rule out sinister pathology
Tonsils	Common and variable. Often symmetrical and may relate to local infection/inflammation (Fig. 8.8)	
Urinary tract	Increased activity within the urinary tract is normal (Fig. 8.2f)	Good hydration and voiding are advised before imaging
Vocal cords	Variable – moderate and symmetrical (Fig. 8.9)	Relates to phonation during uptake period. Unilateral uptake requires further evaluation – may relate to tumour or potentially unilateral vocal cord palsy

PET study should be considered to reduce the false positives. Scanning performed immediately after surgery or biopsy may show falsely increased tracer localisation due to postsurgical inflammation. In addition, infection such as pneumonia, tuberculosis and osteomyelitis leads to false positives in oncology patients [2, 5–9, 12, 13, 16].

Imaging on hybrid PET/CT scanners may lead to misregistration due to differences in breathing patterns and patient movement between CT and PET image acquisitions [5–9]. Patient movement may be avoided by instructing the patient to lie down still during the scan or sometimes by using sedation judiciously in patient with severe pain and in children. Misregistration can be minimised by performing the CT scan during normal expiration. In hybrid PET/CT studies, low-dose CT data is used for attenuation correction of PET data. However, high-density contrast agents or metallic objects may lead to overcorrection if CT data is used for attenuation correction [5]. This leads to falsely increased tracer activity at these sites. Similarly, parts of the brain may show falsely decreased uptake due to under-attenuation correction of PET data if there is patient movement. Reviewing the

Fig. 8.1 Maximum intensity projection (*MIP*) ^{18}F-FDG PET/CT image shows normal physiological tracer distribution in the brain, heart, liver, stomach, bowel and testes and excretion through the kidneys into the urinary bladder. [*It is essential to recognise normal physiological uptake in order to interpret FDG PET images correctly*]

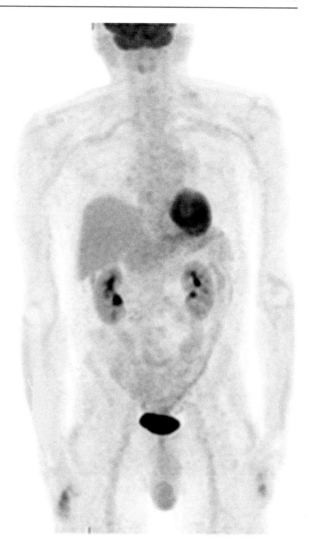

non-attenuation-corrected data is helpful in avoiding such misinterpretation. Another potential problem with low-dose CT for attenuation correction is beam-hardening artefacts, particularly in larger patients. This can lead to inaccurate attenuation correction. However, recently with many centres using diagnostic quality CT in PET/CT studies, this issue is not very frequent. Also, as this is commonly caused by the patient's arms being in the field of view, it can be avoided by placing the arms above the head during imaging. However, if the head and neck are the areas of interest, it is advised to scan the patient in arms-down position. Truncation artefacts are rare but difficult problems with hybrid scanner. These occur in cases where field of view of PET is larger in comparison to CT part [5].

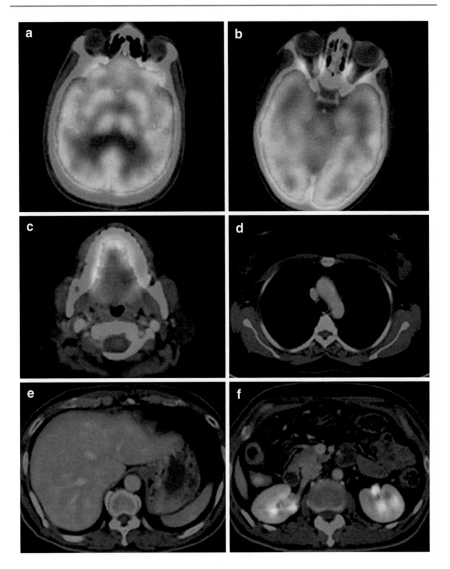

Fig. 8.2 Axial fused PET/CT images from different ^{18}F-FDG PET/CT studies show physiological tracer uptake in the (**a**) brain, (**b**) medial and lateral rectus muscles of orbits, (**c**) tongue, (**d**) breasts, (**e**) liver and collapsed stomach wall, (**f**) kidneys, (**g**) rectum and (**h**) testes

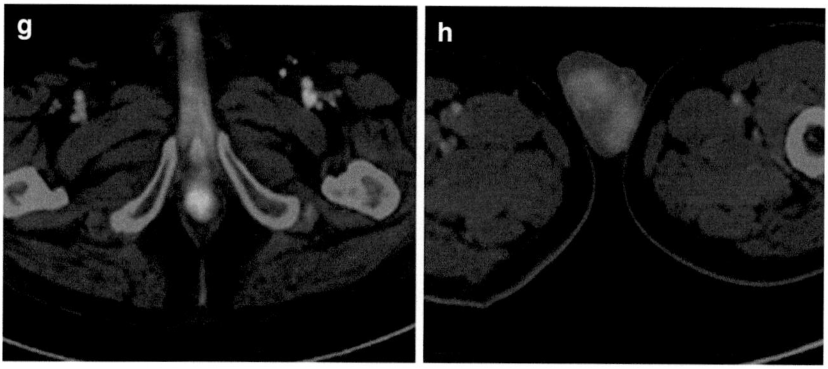

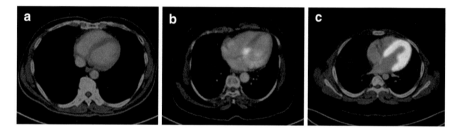

Fig. 8.2 (continued)

Fig. 8.3 18F-FDG PET/CT studies show different patterns of physiological tracer uptake in the myocardium varying from negligible (**a**), segmental (**b**) to diffuse intense uptake (**c**). [*Variable myocardial uptake depends partly on fasting state and may be suppressed by prolonged fast or a low-carbohydrate high-fat diet. In PET cardiac imaging, the main aim is to increase cardiac uptake of FDG by increasing the serum insulin level*]

False positives and false negatives can be countered in 18F-FDG PET studies (Tables 8.3, 8.4 and 8.5). Tracer extravasation leads to false-positive tracer accumulation at the site of injection (Figs. 8.21, 8.22). Knowledge of site of injection is essential in correct interpretation of PET studies. Most of the false positives are due to infectious and inflammatory conditions [5–9]. In addition, many benign tumours may show false-positive 18F-FDG uptake. Similarly some benign tumours show photopenia on PET images (Figs. 8.22, 8.23). Small lesions beyond the resolution

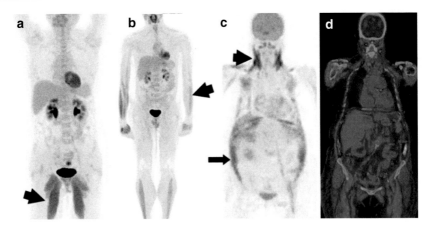

Fig. 8.4 (**a, b**) MIP ¹⁸F-FDG PET image shows uptake in the skeletal muscles (*arrows*) likely due to overuse or muscular strain. This may obscure peripheral primary tumours, e.g. in melanoma. (**c, d**) MIP and coronal fused ¹⁸F-FDG PET/CT images show increased tracer uptake in the respiratory muscles in a patient with breathing difficulty. The diffuse uptake in the abdominal muscles may mimic peritoneal uptake and caution is advised. *[In general, exercising muscles, postexercise, uses glucose (energy substrate); in contrast, resting muscles predominantly uses free fatty acids. Therefore, patients should avoid strenuous/severe exercise for at least a day prior to imaging]*

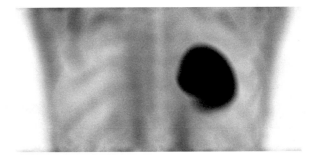

Fig. 8.5 MIP¹⁸F-FDG PET image of a patient for cardiac viability study shows diffuse increased tracer uptake in the muscles due to glucose loading and insulin administration. *[Diffuse muscle uptake can often be seen when the serum insulin level is elevated/increased]*

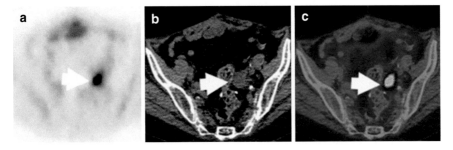

Fig. 8.6 Transaxial PET (**a**), CT (**b**) and fused (**c**) images show. Physiological tracer uptake in the left adnexa (*arrow*) [Adnexal and uterine activity is likely to represent physiological ovarian and uterine uptake in a premenopausal woman and is usually seen in the midcycle. A corpus luteum cyst can present as a "ring" for peripheral uptake in the adnexa. It is important to check the patient's menstrual history. Increased adnexal or uterine uptake in a postmenopausal woman warrants further investigation]

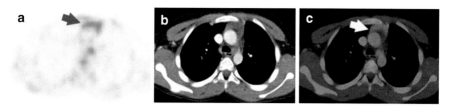

Fig. 8.7 Transaxial PET (**a**), CT (**b**) and fused (**c**) images demonstrate diffuse and homogeneous uptake (*arrow* in **a, c**) in the thymus following chemotherapy due to thymic rebound hyperplasia. [*Thymic tissue is often reactivated post-chemotherapy and is normally seen in children and young adults*]

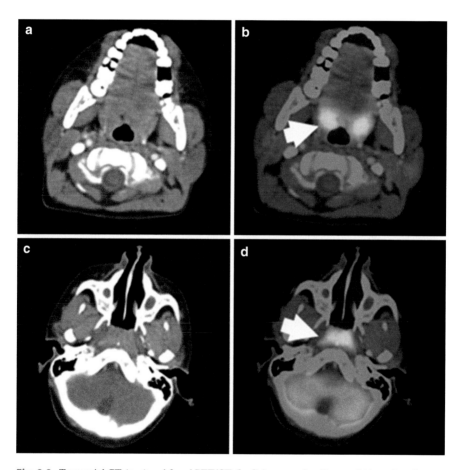

Fig. 8.8 Transaxial CT (**a, c**) and fused PET/CT (**b, d**) images of an 8-year-old boy show intense symmetric uptake in normal tonsils (*arrow* in **b**) and normal adenoids (*arrow* in **d**). [*Intense tracer uptake can be seen in the Waldeyer's ring, especially in children, due to high physiological activity of these lymphatic tissues and peaks at 6–8 years of age*]

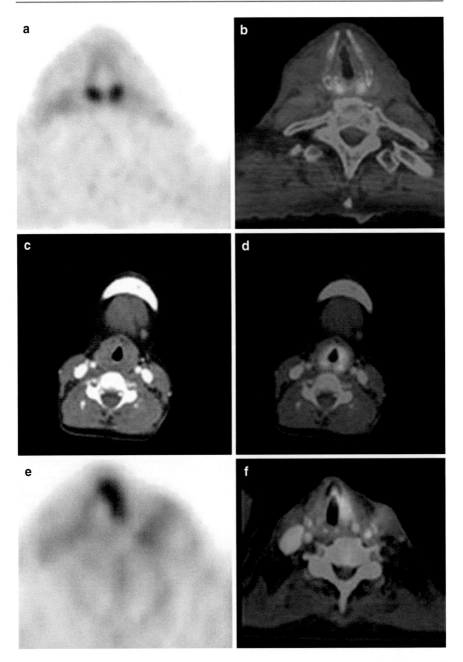

Fig. 8.9 (a, b) Axial ^{18}F-FDG PET and fused PET/CT images show symmetrically increased tracer uptake in the arytenoid muscles. (c, d) Axial CT and fused ^{18}F-FDG PET/CT images show symmetrically increased tracer uptake in the laryngeal muscles. *[This should be minimised in patients with head and neck cancer by maintaining silence after tracer injection.]* (e, f) Axial ^{18}F-FDG PET and fused PET/CT images show asymmetrical increased tracer uptake in the left vocal cord due to recurrent laryngeal nerve palsy on the right. *[When there is asymmetrical uptake in the vocal cords, it is the normal vocal cord that demonstrates increased uptake, and the side with no increased uptake is the side with the nerve palsy]*

Table 8.3 ¹⁸F-FDG scans: false-positive and false-negative tracer uptake in the head/neck regions [5–9, 12, 13, 16]

False positive	False negative
Physiological uptake	Small size
Brown adipose tissue (Fig. 8.10)	Recent high-dose steroid therapy
Inflammatory processes	Hyperglycaemia and hyperinsulinaemia
Postsurgical	Low-grade and well-differentiated tumours
Post-radiotherapy	Misalignment between PET and CT data
Granulomatous disease	(attenuation correction artefacts) (Fig. 8.12)
Post-chemotherapy	
Thyroiditis (Fig. 8.11)	
Benign neoplasms	
Pleomorphic adenomas	
Thyroid adenomas (Fig. 8.11)	
Salivary gland tumours	
Graves' disease (Fig. 8.11)	
Artefacts	
Misalignment between PET and CT data	
(attenuation correction artefacts)	

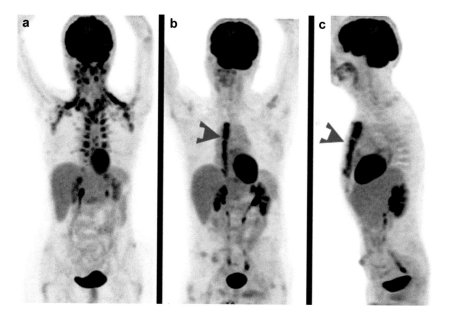

Fig. 8.10 Maximum intensity projection (*MIP*) ¹⁸F-FDG PET images demonstrate (**a**) physiological brown fat uptake in the neck, supraclavicular fossae, mediastinum and suprarenal region (**b, c**) intense tracer uptake in the sternum recent sternotomy (*arrowheads*)

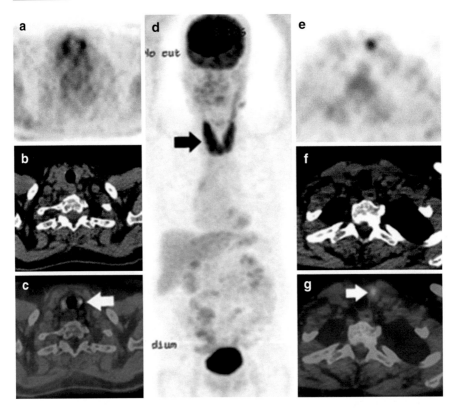

Fig. 8.11 ^{18}F-FDG PET/CT studies (**a, b, c**) transaxial PET, CT and fused images demonstrate diffuse homogenous tracer uptake in a normal size thyroid gland in a patient with known thyroiditis. (**d**) MIP image shows intense diffusely increased uptake (*arrow*) in enlarged thyroid gland in a patient with known Graves' disease; (**e, f, g**) transaxial PET, CT and fused images show focal uptake (*arrow*) in the left thyroid lobe. [*Diffuse uptake is seen in patients with Graves' disease, subacute thyroiditis or Hashimoto's thyroiditis, and thyroid function tests should be recommended; focal uptake in the thyroid can be malignant in approximately one third of patients and should be further evaluated with ultrasound and FNA*]

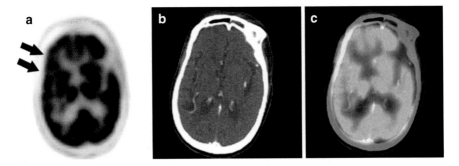

Fig. 8.12 Transaxial ^{18}F-FDG PET (**a**), CT (**b**) and PET/CT (**c**) images of brain show apparent decreased tracer uptake in the right side of brain (arrows) due to head movement leading to under attenuation correction of the right side of brain

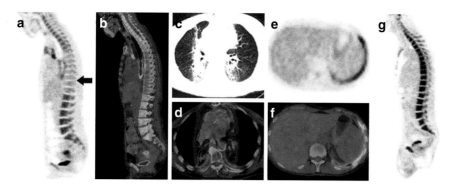

Fig. 8.13 ¹⁸F-FDG PET/CT studies: (**a, b**) sagittal PET and fused PET/CT images show decreased tracer uptake (*arrow* in **a**) in the thoracic vertebrae due to prior radiation therapy to this site; (**c, d**) transaxial CT and fused PET/CT images demonstrate increased uptake in para-mediastinal lung fibrosis after radiotherapy; (**e, f**) transaxial PET and fused PET/CT images demonstrate increased uptake in the left pleura with history of previous talc pleurodesis due to chronic granulomatous reaction. *[Evaluation of mesothelioma is difficult following talc pleurodesis as the resulting increased pleural uptake can persist for several years.]* (**g**) MIP image shows reactive diffuse tracer uptake in the bone marrow following chemotherapy in a lymphoma patient

Table 8.4 ¹⁸F-FDG scans: false-positive and false-negative tracer uptake in the thorax [5–9, 12, 13, 16]

False positive	False negative
Physiological uptake	Small size
Brown adipose tissue (Fig. 8.10)	Recent high-dose steroid therapy
Thymus (children and young adults)	Hyperglycaemia and hyperinsulinaemia
Lactating breast and areolae (Fig. 8.2)	Low-grade and well-differentiated tumours
Skeletal and smooth muscles (Fig. 8.4)	Bronchioalveolar carcinomas
Oesophagus	Lobular carcinomas of the breast
Inflammatory processes	
Postsurgical (Fig. 8.10)	
Post-radiotherapy (Fig. 8.13)	
Post-chemotherapy (Fig. 8.13)	
Infection/inflammation (Fig. 8.14)	
Granulomatous disease (Fig. 8.13)	
Drainage tubes	
Oesophagitis (Fig. 8.14)	
Vasculitis (Fig. 8.14)	
Post-chemotherapy	
Thymic rebound hyperplasia (Fig. 8.7)	
Artefacts	
Misalignment between PET and CT data (attenuation correction artefacts)	

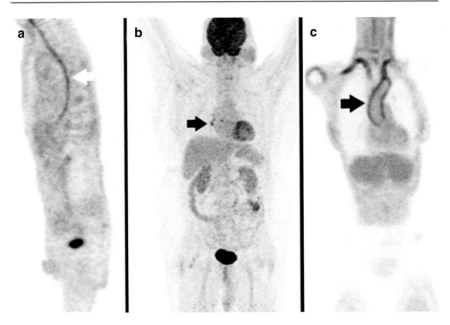

Fig. 8.14 (**a**) MIP[18]F-FDG PET image of a patient shows linear tracer uptake (*arrow*) in through-out the length of oesophagus with no gross morphological changes suggestive of inflammatory activity. (**b**) MIP[18]F-FDG PET image of a follow-up patient of gall bladder carcinoma shows FDG uptake in the mediastinal lymph nodes (*arrow*) with no other sites of significant hypermetabolism likely due to inflammation/infection. (**c**) Coronal PET image of a patient with large-vessel vascu-litis shows diffusely increased FDG uptake in the wall of the aorta and its main branches (*arrow*). *[If a patient is on steroids, this can result in a false-negative PET study in the evaluation of vascu-litis, and ideally steroid therapy needs to be stopped for at least 3 weeks before the PET scan]*

Fig. 8.15 There is diffuse uptake throughout much of the bowel, likely secondary to the patient's metformin use *[In general, patient's metformin use makes image interpretation of bowel pathology difficult]*

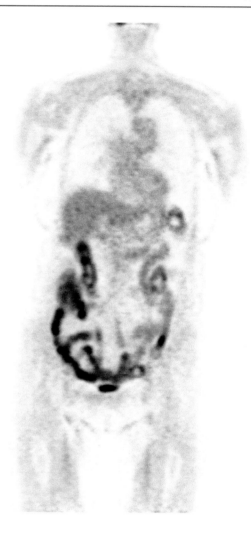

Fig. 8.16 Maximum intensity projection (*MIP*) ¹⁸F-FDG PET image demonstrates intense tracer uptake (*white arrow*) in the anterior abdominal wall at the site of surgical incision in a patient with recent open cholecystectomy. *[Increased uptake after surgery persists for several weeks, and ideally the PET scan should be delayed for at least 6 weeks following surgery.]* There is also increased uptake in the large intestine (*black arrow*)

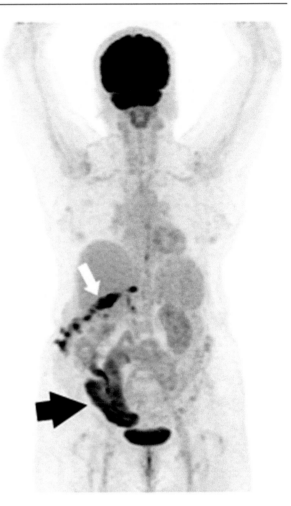

Table 8.5 ^{18}F-FDG scans: false-positive and false-negative tracer uptake in the abdomen and pelvis [5–9, 12, 13, 16]

False positive	False negative
Physiological uptake	Small size
Brown adipose tissue (Fig. 8.10)	Recent high-dose steroid therapy
Skeletal and smooth muscles (Fig. 8.4)	Hyperglycaemia and
Stomach (Fig. 8.2)	hyperinsulinaemia
Bowel (diffuse) (Fig. 8.15)	Low-grade tumours
Kidney and urinary bladder (Fig 8.17)	Well-differentiated carcinomas
Ureters and urethra (Figs. 8.17, 8.18 and 8.19)	Hepatocellular carcinoma
Uterus during menses or corpus luteum cyst (Fig. 8.6)	Neuroendocrine tumours
Ileostomy loop (Fig. 8.17)	Mucous secreting tumours
Inflammatory processes	Prostate carcinoma
Drainage tubes	
Postsurgical (Fig. 8.16)	
Post-radiotherapy	
Post-chemotherapy	
Inflammatory bowel disease	
Cholecystitis	
Pancreatitis	
Psoas abscess	
Benign neoplasms	
Adrenal adenoma	
Ovarian cystadenoma	
Uterine fibroid (Fig. 8.20)	
Artefacts	
Misalignment between PET and CT data (attenuation correction artefacts) (Fig. 8.21)	

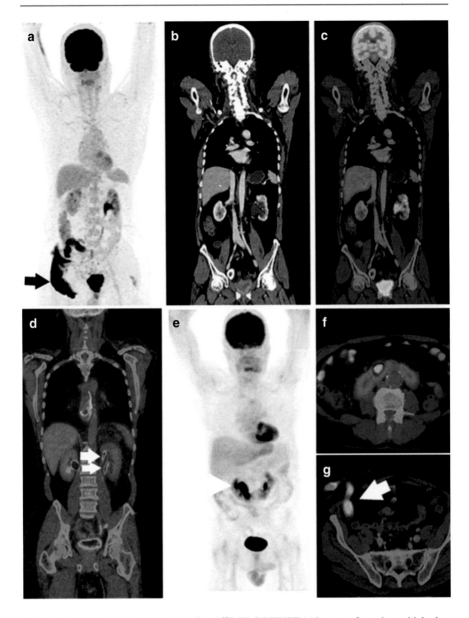

Fig. 8.17 MIP (**a**), coronal CT (**b**) and fused ^{18}F-FDG PET/CT (**c**) images of a patient with hydronephrosis of the left kidney show tracer retention in the dilated pelvicalyceal system of the left kidney. (**a, g**) Intense physiological tracer uptake is also noted in the ileostomy loop (*arrow*). Coronal fused ^{18}F-FDG PET/CT image (**d**) of a patient with duplex left kidney shows tracer uptake in two ureters (*arrows*), which may be mistaken as a lymph node in transaxial images. MIP (**e**) and transaxial fused ^{18}F-FDG PET/CT (**f**) images of a patient with horseshoe kidney show tracer activity within the fused kidneys in the midline of the abdomen

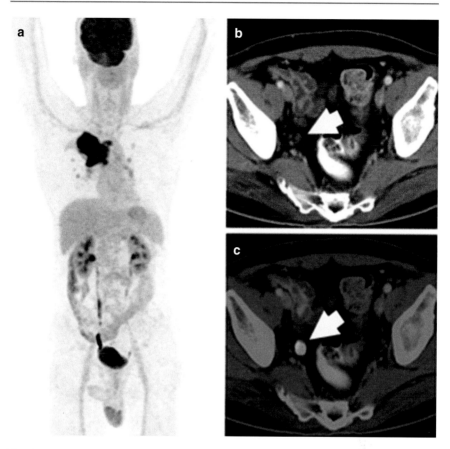

Fig. 8.18 Tracer uptake in the dilated ureter may mimic a lymph node (*arrows* in **b, c**). *[Correlation of tracer activity on the MIP image (**a**) and following the ureter on transaxial images are helpful]*

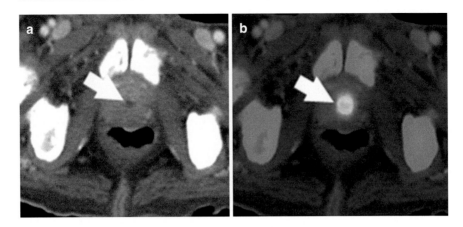

Fig. 8.19 Physiological intense focal urinary tracer activity in the prostatic urethra (*arrows* in **a**, **b**) in a patient with adenocarcinoma of the prostate following transurethral resection of the prostate. [*Most prostate cancers are not FDG avid; however approximately 10–15% of incidental focal prostate uptake is related to malignancy, and if seen, biochemical evaluation with serum PSA is advised*]

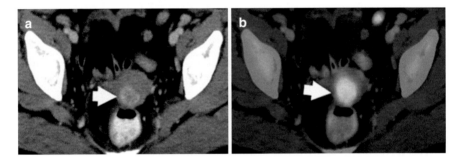

Fig. 8.20 Intense tracer uptake is seen in an enhancing soft tissue lesion in the uterine wall (*arrows* in **a**, **b**) suggestive of fibroid. [*Any increased uptake in the uterus in a postmenopausal woman should be investigated, and an ultrasound is advised in the first instance*]

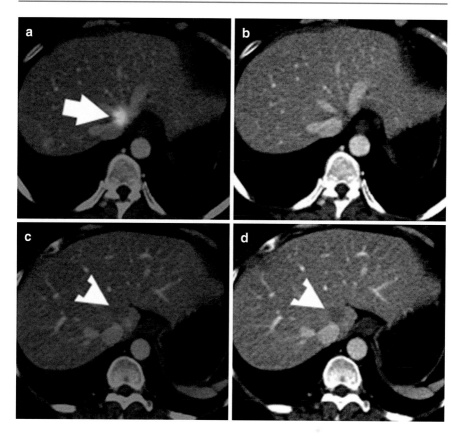

Fig. 8.21 Misregistration: Transaxial fused ^{18}F-FDG PET/CT and CT images show a hypodense hepatic lesion (*arrowhead* in **c, d**) that has been misplaced to slightly higher level during PET image acquisition (*arrow* in **a**) due to differences in breathing patterns between CT and PET image acquisitions. Note there is no lesion on CT image (**b**) corresponding to apparent site of tracer uptake on fused image (*arrow* in **a**). *[In general, motion artefacts, reconstruction artefacts and noise are usually self-evident in most cases]*

Fig. 8.22 MIP ^{18}F-FDG
PET image shows tracer
extravasation at the site of
injection (*arrows*).*[A local
view of the extravasation
site is often undertaken to
establish what proportion
of the administered activity
remains at the
extravasation site. The
SUV measurements will
also be affected]*

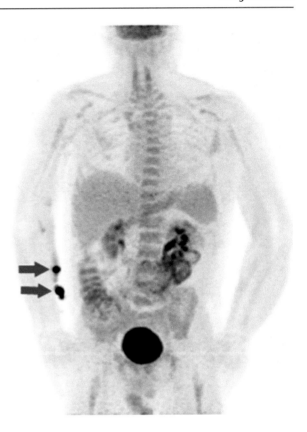

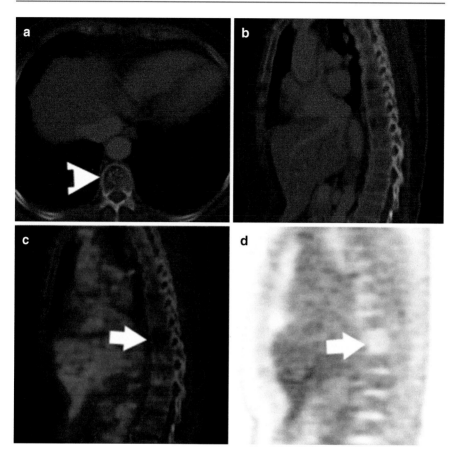

Fig. 8.23 Sagittal CT, fused and PET (**b**, **c**, **d**) images show. Focal photopenia (*arrows* in **c**, **d**) in a vertebral haemangioma showing "polka-dot appearance" on corresponding transaxial CT image (*arrowhead* in **a**). *[Vertebral haemangiomata can be "hot" or "cold" on FDG PET imaging]*

of PET scanners usually do not show ¹⁸F-FDG uptake. Further, many cancers, such as lung carcinoid, are generally negative of ¹⁸F-FDG PET studies. These false interpretations can be reduced by including CT findings in the PET/CT reports.

Conclusions

It is vital to recognise the normal variants and artefacts for accurate interpretation of ¹⁸F-FDG PET/CT studies. Furthermore, recognising false positives and false negatives is equally important for correct interpretation of PET/CT findings.

Key Points
- ^{18}F-FDG is transported into cells through glucose transporters and phosphorylated by enzyme hexokinase to ^{18}F-FDG-6-phosphate.
- ^{18}F-FDG is accumulated in malignant tissues more avidly than within the normal tissues.
- ^{18}F-FDG PET/CT scans often show variable degree of physiological tracer uptake is noted in various organs.
- Recognition of physiological tracer distribution is essential in avoiding wrong image interpretation.
- It is vital to recognise normal variants and artefacts to avoid misinterpretation.
- Misregistration is noted due to differences in breathing patterns and patient movement between CT and PET image acquisitions. It is vital to recognise misregistration to avoid misinterpretation.
- False positives and false negatives can be countered in ^{18}F-FDG PET studies.
- ^{18}F-FDG uptake is known to occur in inflammation, infection and healing tissues.
- ^{18}F-FDG PET study immediately after chemotherapy and radiotherapy may introduce false-positive findings.
- Recognising false positives and false negatives is important for accurate reporting.

Acknowledgements The authors would like to thanks to Dr Nerriman, Dr Riyamma and Dr Halsey for contributing images for the chapter on PET/CT Imaging: Normal Variants, Pitfalls and Artefacts.

References

1. Agrawal K, Mittal BR, Bansal D, et al. Role of F-18 FDG PET/CT in assessing bone marrow involvement in pediatric Hodgkin's lymphoma. Ann Nucl Med. 2013;27(2):146–51.
2. Mittal BR, Agrawal K. FDG-PET in tuberculosis. Curr Mol Imaging. 2014;3(3):211–5.
3. Cook GJ, Fogelman I, Maisey MN. Normal physiological and benign pathological variants of ^{18}F-FDG PET scanning: potential for error in interpretation. Semin Nucl Med. 1996;26:308–14.
4. Cook GJ, Maisey MN, Fogelman I. Normal variants, artefacts and interpretative pitfalls in PET imaging with ^{18}F-fluoro-2-deoxyglucose and carbon-11 methionine. Eur J Nucl Med. 1999;26:1363–78.
5. Cook GJ, Wegner EA, Fogelman I. Pitfalls and artifacts in 18 FDG PET and PET/CT oncologic imaging. Semin Nucl Med. 2004;34:122–33.
6. Culverwell AD, Scarsbrook AF, Chowdhury FU. False-positive uptake on 2-[^{18}F]-fluoro-2-deoxy-D-glucose (FDG) positron-emission tomography/computed tomography (PET/CT) in oncological imaging. Clin Radiol. 2011;66:366–82.
7. Shreve PD, Anzai Y, Wahl RL. Pitfalls in oncologic diagnosis with FDG PET imaging: physiologic and benign variants. Radiographics. 1999;19:61–77.

8. Delbeke D, Coleman RE, Guiberteau MJ, et al. Procedure guideline for tumour imaging with ¹⁸F-FDG PET/CT 1.0. J Nucl Med. 2006;47:885–95.
9. Boellaard R, O'Doherty MJ, Weber WA, et al. FDG PET and PET/CT: EANM procedure guidelines for tumour PET imaging: version 1.0. Eur J Nucl Med Mol Imaging. 2010;37:181–200.
10. Segall G, Delbeke D, Stabin MG, et al. SNM practice guideline for sodium 18F-fluoride PET/CT bone scans 1.0. J Nucl Med. 2010;51:1813–20.
11. Juweid ME, Cheson BD. Positron-emission tomography and assessment of cancer therapy. N Engl J Med. 2006;354:496–507.
12. Gorospe L, Raman S, Echeveste J, et al. Whole-body PET/CT: spectrum of physiological variants, artifacts and interpretative pitfalls in cancer patients. Nucl Med Commun. 2005;26:671–87.
13. Shammas A, Lim R, Charron M. Pediatric FDG PET/CT: physiologic uptake, normal variants, and benign conditions. Radiographics. 2009;29:1467–86.
14. Harisankar CN, Mittal BR, Agrawal KL, et al. Utility of high fat and low carbohydrate diet in suppressing myocardial FDG uptake. J Nucl Cardiol. 2011;18:926–36.
15. Agrawal K, Weaver J, Ngu R, et al. Clinical significance of patterns of incidental thyroid uptake at (18)F-FDG PET/CT. Clin Radiol. 2015;70(5):536–43.
16. Corrigan AJ, Schleyer PJ, Cook GJ. Pitfalls and artifacts in the use of PET/CT in oncology imaging. Semin Nucl Med. 2015;45(6):481–99.

PET/CT in Gynaecological Malignancies

9

Sairah R. Khan and Tara Barwick

Contents

S.R. Khan
Department of Radiology, Imperial College Healthcare NHS Trust, Charing Cross Hospital,
London, UK
e-mail: sairah.khan@imperial.nhs.uk

T. Barwick (✉)
Imperial College Healthcare NHS Trust, London, UK

Department of Surgery and Cancer, Imperial College, London, UK
e-mail: tara.barwick@imperial.nhs.uk

© Springer International Publishing Switzerland 2016
T. Barwick, A. Rockall (eds.), *PET/CT in Gynecological Cancers*,
Clinicians' Guides to Radionuclide Hybrid Imaging, DOI 10.1007/978-3-319-29249-6_9

9.1   Introduction

Over the past decade, there is increasing evidence supporting the use of FDG PET/CT for several specific indications in gynaecological malignancies. The primary indications are staging of locally advanced cervical cancer prior to chemoradiation therapy, prior to pelvic exenteration and prior to salvage radiotherapy or surgery for any gynaecological malignancy in what is thought to be single-site disease on conventional workup. It is also beneficial in the assessment of suspected relapse ovarian cancer when conventional imaging is negative.

There is less defined clinical impact of the role of FDG PET/CT in vulval and vaginal malignancies which are relatively rare and have not been discussed in this guide due to space limitations.

9.2   Technical Aspects and Limitations of PET/CT Specific to Gynaecological Malignancies

Knowledge of the common physiologic patterns of FDG uptake is essential to reduce interpretation pitfalls. There may be FDG uptake in normal ovaries during menstruation and ovulation and increased endometrial activity during menstruation. The typical appearance of physiologic uptake in the ovary is spherical with smooth margins or sometimes a rim of activity with a photopenic centre, and on CT it may appear as a small rim-enhancing cyst. Physiologic endometrial activity in a premenopausal woman is typically diffuse and uniform. Conversely focal uterine or ovarian activity in a postmenopausal woman requires investigation with transvaginal ultrasound to exclude pathology (Fig. 9.1).

Uterine fibroids, hydrosalpinges and benign endometriotic cysts may also be metabolically active on PET imaging and mimic pathology. Tracer hold-up in the ureters may mimic nodal disease. In addition, in postsurgical cases where the anatomy is distorted, tracer retention in the bladder and/or complications such as vesico-vaginal fistulas can mask or mimic disease. Some necrotic, mucinous, cystic or low-grade tumours may have low-level glucose metabolism and be less readily detected by FDG PET/CT.

The limited spatial resolution of PET means that it has lower utility for detecting small lesions and in diagnosing primary lesions that may be occult on the PET study. In addition, respiratory motion next to the hemidiaphragms and related to physiologic bowel movement may hamper the assessment of small-volume peritoneal/serosal disease. These pitfalls are summarised in Table 9.1.

Good techniques include emptying the bladder immediately prior to the scan and scanning in the caudo-cranial direction so the pelvis is imaged first. The administration of diuretics and butylscopolamine has been reported to help, but is not typically used routinely. Depending on local practice, if applicable, the patient may be scanned on a flatbed in the radiotherapy-planning position to facilitate PET-guided radiotherapy planning.

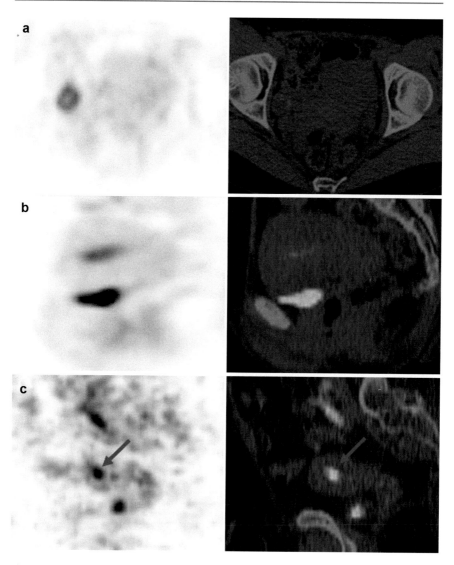

Fig. 9.1 PET and fused axial images show (**a**) typical appearance of a corpus luteum cyst with a rim of peripheral activity, (**b**) linear activity in the endometrium in a typical configuration consistent with physiologic uptake during menstruation. (**c**) Incidental focal intense endometrial activity (*red arrow*) in a postmenopausal woman being investigated for a solitary pulmonary nodule. Transvaginal ultrasound (not shown) demonstrated increased endometrial thickness of 15 mm histopathology revealed endometrial carcinoma

Table 9.1 Limitations and pitfalls related to gynaecological cancer

Potential false positives	Potential false negatives
Physiologic activity in ovaries and endometrium during ovulation/menstruation	Some necrotic, mucinous, cystic or low-grade tumours may be low-level active and less readily detected
Some benign lesions such as uterine fibroids and benign endometriosis cysts can be metabolically active	Limited spatial resolution of PET can miss small-volume disease especially small-volume peritoneal disease and small lymph nodes
Focal ureteric activity or focal bladder activity can mimic disease	Respiratory motion artefact near hemidiaphragms may miss sub-diaphragmatic peritoneal disease
Vesico-vaginal fistulas may also limit disease evaluation	

9.3 Cervical Cancer

9.3.1 Staging Primary Cervical Cancer

There is no role for FDG PET/CT in screening for cervical cancer, detection of the primary tumour or accurate T staging of the primary tumour, due to the limited spatial resolution such that some small tumours may be occult on the PET. Furthermore, FDG PET cannot differentiate between post-cone biopsy inflammation and residual tumour. As detailed in Chap. 4, pelvic MRI is the best modality for assessing the primary tumour and involvement of local structures such as the parametrium.

Nodal involvement, although not included in the FIGO staging, is an important prognostic marker and guides therapeutic management. There is no routine use for FDG PET/CT in the nodal staging of early stage cervical cancer. This group of patients have a very low incidence of nodal disease, and if present it may be small volume/microscopic and below the resolution of PET. Thus the performance of PET for nodal staging of early stage cervical cancer is disappointing.

However, in locally advanced cervical tumours, which are typically treated by brachytherapy, external beam radiotherapy to the pelvis and concurrent chemotherapy (Chap. 3), the diagnostic performance of FDG PET/CT is better than standard MRI/CT [2, 22].

Perhaps more important is the detection of retroperitoneal nodal disease, which occurs in 15–30 % of patients with locally advanced cervical cancer, as this may be amenable to extended field radiotherapy (Fig. 9.2) or distant disease, for example, supraclavicular nodes (Fig. 9.3). In a meta-analysis of PET in the detection of para-aortic nodal disease, the overall sensitivity was low and heterogenous but the specificity was high, and there was a trend to increasing sensitivity with higher prevalence of nodal disease [8]. In other words, PET is more reliable in patients who have a higher pre-test probability of nodal disease.

Based on evidence for staging of cervical cancers, in particular improved N and M staging, FDG PET/CT is recommended by the National Comprehensive Cancer

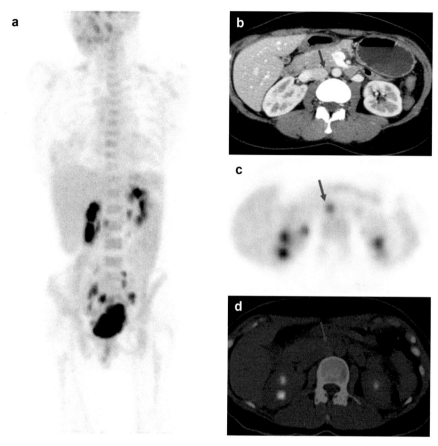

Fig. 9.2 A 38-year-old patient with stage IIIa cervical cancer prior to chemoradiation therapy. The MIP (**a**), transaxial PET and fused images (**c, d**) demonstrate metabolically active pelvic lymph nodes and aortocaval lymph nodes (*red arrows*). The retroperitoneal nodes were not appreciated on the contrast-enhanced staging CT (**b**) examination due to their small size

Network (NCCN), Royal College of Radiologist (RCR) and Scottish Intercollegiate Guidelines Network (SIGN) guidelines for assessment of locally advanced cervical cancer (>1B1) prior to chemoradiation therapy [13, 14, 20].

9.3.2 Recurrence

There is no definitive evidence to support the routine use of FDG PET/CT in the follow-up of patients post cervical cancer treatment, although some groups advocate a routine FDG PET/CT 3 months post chemoradiation therapy in cases of locally advanced cervical cancer particularly as a prognostic marker for overall outcome [18, 19]. The SIGN guidelines acknowledge that the

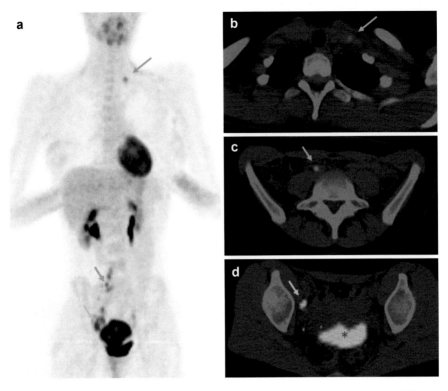

Fig. 9.3 A 46-year-old patient with newly diagnosed stage IB 2 cervical cancer. PET/CT performed to assess the extent of disease. The MIP (**a**) and fused images (**b**, **c** and **d**) demonstrate the large metabolically active cervical tumour (*red star*) with the right pelvic side wall lymph nodes (*yellow arrows*). In addition, PET/CT demonstrated small right common iliac nodes (*green arrows*) and distant disease with a left supraclavicular node (*blue arrows*)

evidence for post-treatment surveillance is inconsistent but suggest that a PET/CT 9 months post-treatment may be helpful in patients who have had chemoradiation therapy and that a PET/CT should also be performed in cases of recurrence in whom salvage therapy (pelvic exenteration or radiotherapy) is being considered, in order to rule out distant disease [20]. The UK RCR guidelines suggest PET/CT should be used in patients being considered for exenterative surgery and for suspected recurrence when other imaging is equivocal [14]. A recent systematic review of PET/CT in recurrent cervical cancer suggested that the routine addition of PET/CT to standard diagnostic strategy (clinical examination, MRI and/or CT scan) although more accurate was not felt to be cost-effective; however it recognised the lack of good quality evidence in this scenario [12]. However, in patients with pelvic recurrence thought suitable for pelvic exenteration on conventional workup with pelvic MRI and CT chest, abdomen and pelvis, FDG PET/CT may detect distant disease beyond the pelvis and avoid futile surgery [5, 20].

9.4 Endometrial Cancer

9.4.1 Primary Staging of Endometrial Cancer

As mentioned in Chap. 3, endometrial cancers are primarily staged and treated by surgery, typically total abdominal hysterectomy. The benefits of surgical lymphadenectomy are controversial and practice varies. MRI is the modality of choice for staging of the primary tumour. However, there is a need for a non-invasive assessment of nodal disease prior to surgery. The results of FDG PET/CT in the nodal staging of endometrial cancers have been disappointing to date with overall suboptimal sensitivity but relatively high specificity. A recent meta-analysis of 16 studies of FDG PET/CT in endometrial cancer reported pooled sensitivity and specificity of 72.3 and 92.9 %, respectively, for nodal staging and 95.7 and 95.4 % for distant metastases [7]. The high specificity and positive predictive value mean of FDG PET/CT may be useful in selected cases such as equivocal retroperitoneal nodes or distant disease on conventional workup, or in poor surgical candidates. In the UK, there is currently a multicentre study [11] investigating the diagnostic performance of diffusion-weighted MRI, FDG PET/CT and fluoroethycholine PET/CT in the nodal staging of surgically staged high-risk endometrial and cervical cancers which should provide further information regarding the role of FDG PET/CT in this setting [11].

9.4.2 Recurrence

There is no role for FDG PET/CT in the routine follow-up/surveillance of endometrial cancer patients. However, FDG PET/CT can be useful prior to salvage radiotherapy or surgery by ensuring there is no disease beyond the surgical/radiotherapy field (Fig. 9.4). A recent meta-analysis of 11 studies of FDG PET in recurrent endometrial cancer patients reported the treatment plan changed in 22–35 % of the studied patients [6].

9.5 Ovarian Cancer

9.5.1 Characterisation of Adnexal Masses

There is no routine role for PET/CT in the characterisation of adnexal masses. Although malignant lesions tend to be more metabolically active than benign lesion, there is overlap in the level of metabolic activity particularly between benign lesions and borderline tumours [10]. False negatives have been reported with borderline and low-grade tumours and false positives in hydrosalpinges, endometriosis and pedunculated fibroids. Transvaginal ultrasound +/− MRI are the modalities of choice for adnexal mass characterisation [21] (Chap. 4).

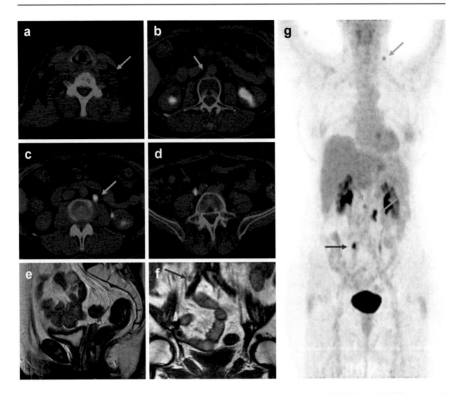

Fig. 9.4 A 74-year-old patient with previous endometrial cancer treated with TAH and BSO presented with PV bleeding. MRI pelvis (**e**) revealed vaginal recurrence (*red arrow*). PET/CT (fused images **a–d**, MIP **g**) was performed to see if suitable for pelvic exenterative surgery. The FDG PET/CT revealed a left supraclavicular node (**a**, **g** *yellow arrow*), small retroperitoneal nodes (**b**, **c**, **g** *green* and *blue arrows*) and a right common iliac node (**d**, **g** *purple arrow*) in retrospect on the MRI (**f**) but tiny

9.5.2 Primary Staging

Ovarian cancer typically spreads to local lymph nodes, the peritoneum by lymphatic channels or less frequently haematogenous dissemination to distant organs. The imaging staging is primarily by CECT (Chap. 4). Integrated FDG PET/CT/contrast-enhanced CT has been reported to be more accurate than CECT alone in predicting the surgical staging [9]. However, false negatives may occur typically with small nodes/peritoneal nodules (<7 mm) or cystic/mucinous lesions. Currently, there is insufficient evidence that either PET/CT or integrated PET/CECT gives significant additional benefit over CECT alone in terms of patient outcome and cost-effectiveness to support their routine use [12].

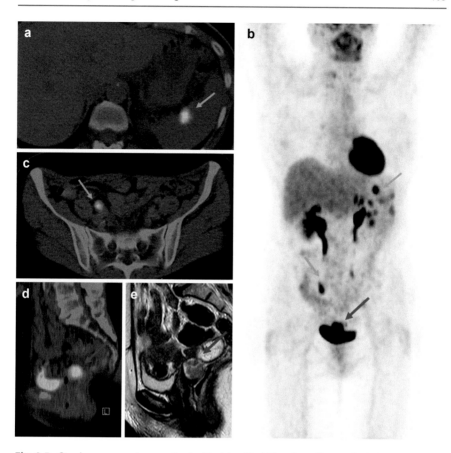

Fig. 9.5 Ovarian cancer relapse patient with rising Ca-125 and a solitary splenic hilar peritoneal deposit on CECT. FDG PET/CT (fused images **a**, **c** and **d**, MIP **b**) prior to surgery demonstrated the metabolically active splenic deposit (**a**, **b**, *blue arrows*) but in addition revealed a small right common iliac lymph node (**b**, **c**, *green arrows*) which was not appreciated on the initial restaging CECT. In addition there was a focal intense activity at the vaginal vault (**b**, **d**, *red arrows*). This was confirmed on subsequent MRI to be recurrence (**e**), and the patient management was changed to chemotherapy rather than surgery

9.5.3 Ovarian Cancer Relapse

FDG PET/CT should not be used in routine post therapy surveillance of ovarian cancer patients. However, there is evidence to support the use of PET/CT in the scenario of suspected relapse with rising tumour markers particularly when conventional imaging with CECT and MRI is negative or equivocal (Fig. 9.5). In a meta-analysis of 34

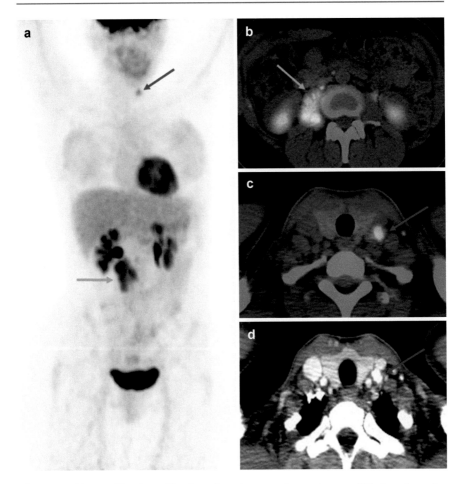

Fig. 9.6 A 52-year-old patient with relapsed mucinous ovarian carcinoma within the retroperitoneum thought to be single site on CECT and potentially suitable for salvage radiotherapy. The pre radiotherapy FDG PET/CT (MIP **a**, fused images **b**, **c**) demonstrated the metabolically active retroperitoneal disease (**a**, **b**, *green arrows*). In addition there was a tiny left supraclavicular node (**a**, **c**, *red arrows*) not appreciated on the CECT as it was calcified (**d** CECT *red arrow*)

studies by Gu et al., the area under the receiver operating curve was 0.92 for CA-125, 0.96 for PET/CT, 0.88 for CECT and 0.8 for MRI in the detection of ovarian cancer recurrence [4]. Ca-125 had the highest pooled specificity (93 %) and PET/CT has the highest pooled sensitivity (91 %). A prospective multicentre study assessing the impact of PET/CT in recurrent ovarian cancer patients reported PET/CT affected management in 60 % (49 % high, 11 % medium impact) [3].

In addition FDG PET/CT may be useful in cases thought to be localised recurrence and potentially amenable to salvage surgery or radiotherapy (Fig. 9.6).

9.6   Future Roles

9.6.1   Radiotherapy Planning

Individualised treatment planning is gaining interest. PET/CT data may be incorporated into radiotherapy planning by providing information about staging and viable tumour tissue and is important for intensity-modulated radiation therapy (IMRT). PET/CT-guided IMRT may permit higher doses of radiation to the primary tumour and to the involved nodal disease whilst minimising treatment-related toxicity [17].

9.6.2   Prognostic Information

Various PET-derived prognostic factors at baseline, early during therapy and at 3 months post completion of chemoradiation therapy have been shown to predict outcome in cases of locally advanced cervical cancer [1]. It is possible in the future these prognostic factors may help tailor therapy and/or select patients for clinical trials. In endometrial cancers, the primary tumour preoperative SUV max is higher in patients with high FIGO stages and nodal metastases and could potentially help select patients for adjuvant therapy [23].

9.6.3   Early Response Assessment

There is evidence that FDG PET/CT may detect response early during chemoradiation therapy for cervical cancer [18] and chemotherapy for ovarian cancer [15]. However, further clinical trials would have to validate defined FDG/PET criteria with which treatment can be safely changed [16].

9.6.4   Technical Advances

Hybrid PET/MR systems have recently become available primarily as a research tool. PET/MR might improve the diagnostic performance of PET/CT based on the major strengths of MR such as superb soft tissue contrast and spatial resolution, particularly for pelvic malignancies.

9.6.5   New Tracers

The use of new more specific tracers and analysis of information derived from a combination of tracers and/or combining functional MRI data with PET data may be useful in therapeutic planning. For example, hypoxic tracers may help select patients for a radiotherapy boost or guide IMRT.

Table 9.2 Summary of main current and potential future indications of FDG PET/CT in gynaecological malignancies

Current indications FDG PET/CT

Staging of locally advanced cervical cancer (>1B1) prior to CRT

Prior to pelvic exenteration (recurrent cervical/endometrial cancers) when conventional workup with pelvic MRI/CT scan is equivocal or negative for extra-pelvic disease

Suspected ovarian cancer relapse when conventional workup is negative/equivocal

Recurrent disease (cervical/ovarian/endometrial) prior to salvage radiotherapy or surgery for what is thought to be single-site disease on conventional workup with pelvic MRI and CECT

Potential future applications

Prognostic information (tumour SUV max), TGV may target patients for neoadjuvant/adjuvant therapy in the clinical trial scenario

Early response assessment during CRT/chemotherapy

Technical advances with PET/MRI

New tracers

9.7   Summary

Table 9.2 summarises the main current indications for FDG PET/CT in gynaecological cancers and potential future roles.

Key Points
- Knowledge of the common physiologic patterns of FDG uptake is essential to reduce interpretation pitfalls.
- FDG uptake in normal ovaries during menstruation and ovulation and increased endometrial activity during menstruation.
- Focal uterine or ovarian activity in a postmenopausal woman requires investigation with transvaginal ultrasound to exclude pathology.
- Uterine fibroids, hydrosalpinges and benign endometriotic cysts may also be metabolically active on PET imaging and mimic pathology.
- Necrotic, mucinous, cystic or low-grade tumours may have low-level glucose metabolism and be less readily detected by FDG PET/CT.
- The limited spatial resolution of PET means that it has lower utility for detecting small lesions and in diagnosing primary lesions that may be occult on the PET study.

Cervical Cancer
- Staging primary cervical cancer: There is no role for FDG PET/CT in screening for cervical cancer, detection of the primary tumour or accurate T staging of the primary tumour.
- There is no routine use for FDG PET/CT in the nodal staging of early stage cervical cancer.

- In locally advanced cervical tumours (typically treated by brachytherapy, external beam radiotherapy to the pelvis and concurrent chemotherapy), the diagnostic performance of FDG PET/CT is better than standard MRI/CT.
- PET is more reliable in detection of retroperitoneal nodal disease, in patients with locally advanced cervical cancer.
- FDG PET/CT is recommended by the National Comprehensive Cancer Network (NCCN), Royal College of Radiologist and Scottish Intercollegiate Guidelines Network (SIGN) guidelines for assessment of locally advanced cervical cancer (>1B1) prior to chemoradiation therapy.
- Recurrence: There is no definitive evidence to support the routine use of FDG PET/CT in the follow-up of patients following cervical cancer treatment.
- The UK RCR guidelines suggest PET/CT should be used in patients being considered for exenterative surgery and for suspected recurrence when other imaging is equivocal.

Endometrial Cancer
- Primary staging of endometrial cancer: MRI is the modality of choice for staging of the primary tumour. However, there is a need for a non-invasive assessment of nodal disease prior to surgery.
- The results of FDG PET/CT in the nodal staging of endometrial cancers have been disappointing to date.
- Recurrence: There is no role for FDG PET/CT in the routine follow-up/ surveillance of endometrial cancer patients. However, FDG PET/CT can be useful prior to salvage radiotherapy or surgery by ensuring there is no disease without the surgical/radiotherapy field.

Ovarian Cancer
- Characterisation of adnexal masses: There is no routine role for PET/CT in the characterisation of adnexal masses. Transvaginal ultrasound +/– MRI are the modalities of choice for adnexal mass characterisation
- Primary staging: Integrated FDG PET/CT/contrast-enhanced CT has been reported to be more accurate than CECT alone in predicting the surgical staging.
- There is insufficient evidence that either PET/CT or integrated PET/CECT gives significant additional benefit over CECT alone in terms of patient outcome and cost-effectiveness to support their routine use.
- Ovarian cancer relapse: FDG PET/CT should not be used in routine post therapy surveillance of ovarian cancer patients. However, there is evidence to support the use of PET/CT in the scenario of suspected relapse with rising tumour markers particularly when conventional imaging with CECT and MRI is negative or equivocal.
- FDG PET/CT may be useful in cases thought to be localised recurrence and potentially amenable to salvage surgery or radiotherapy.

References

1. Barwick TD, Taylor A, Rockall A. Functional imaging to predict tumor response in locally advanced cervical cancer. Curr Oncol Rep. 2013;15(6):549–58.
2. Choi HJ, Ju W, Myung SK, Kim Y. Diagnostic performance of computer tomography, magnetic resonance imaging, and positron emission tomography or positron emission tomography/computer tomography for detection of metastatic lymph nodes in patients with cervical cancer: meta-analysis. Cancer Sci. 2010;101(6):1471–9.
3. Fulham MJ, Carter J, Baldey A, Hicks RJ, Ramshaw JE, Gibson M. The impact of PET-CT in suspected recurrent ovarian cancer: a prospective multi-centre study as part of the Australian PET data collection project. Gynecol Oncol. 2009;112(3):462–8.
4. Gu P, Pan LL, Wu SQ, Sun L, Huang G. CA 125, PET alone, PET-CT, CT and MRI in diagnosing recurrent ovarian carcinoma: a systematic review and meta-analysis. Eur J Radiol. 2009; 71(1):164–74.
5. Husain A, Akhurst T, Larson S, Alektiar K, Barakat RR, Chi DS. A prospective study of the accuracy of 18Fluorodeoxyglucose positron emission tomography (18FDG PET) in identifying sites of metastasis prior to pelvic exenteration. Gynecol Oncol. 2007;106(1):177–80.
6. Kadkhodayan S, Shahriari S, Treglia G, Yousefi Z, Sadeghi R. Accuracy of 18-F-FDG PET imaging in the follow up of endometrial cancer patients: systematic review and meta-analysis of the literature. Gynecol Oncol. 2013;128(2):397–404.
7. Kakhki VR, Shahriari S, Treglia G, Hasanzadeh M, Zakavi SR, Yousefi Z, Kadkhodayan S, Sadeghi R. Diagnostic performance of fluorine 18 fluorodeoxyglucose positron emission tomography imaging for detection of primary lesion and staging of endometrial cancer patients: systematic review and meta-analysis of the literature. Int J Gynecol Cancer. 2013; 23(9):1536–43.
8. Kang S, Kim SK, Chung DC, Seo SS, Kim JY, Nam BH, Park SY. Diagnostic value of (18) F-FDG PET for evaluation of paraaortic nodal metastasis in patients with cervical carcinoma: a metaanalysis. J Nucl Med. 2010;51(3):360–7.
9. Kitajima K, Murakami K, Yamasaki E, Kaji Y, Fukasawa I, Inaba N, Sugimura K. Diagnostic accuracy of integrated FDG-PET/contrast-enhanced CT in staging ovarian cancer: comparison with enhanced CT. Eur J Nucl Med Mol Imaging. 2008;35(10):1912–20.
10. Kitajima K, Suzuki K, Senda M, Kita M, Nakamoto Y, Onishi Y, Maeda T, Yoshikawa T, Ohno Y, Sugimura K. FDG-PET/CT for diagnosis of primary ovarian cancer. Nucl Med Commun. 2011;32(7):549–53.
11. MAPPING study. Available at http://www.cancerresearchuk.org/cancer-help/trials/a-study-comparing-mri-scan-pet-ct-scan-cervical-womb-cancer-mapping.
12. Meads C, Auguste P, Davenport C, Malysiak S, Sundar S, Kowalska M, Zapalska A, Guest P, Thangaratinam S, Martin-Hirsch P, Borowiack E, Barton P, Roberts T, Khan K. Positron emission tomography/computerised tomography imaging in detecting and managing recurrent cervical cancer: systematic review of evidence, elicitation of subjective probabilities and economic modelling. Health Technol Assess. 2013;17(12):1–323.
13. National Comprehensive Cancer Network (NCCN) guidelines for cervical cancer. 2010. Available at http://www.nccn.org/professionals/physician_gls/pdf/cervical.pdf.
14. Royal College of Radiologists. RCR PET guidelines. 2012. Available at http://www.rcr.ac.uk/docs/radiology/pdf/BFCR(12)3_PETCT.pdf.
15. Rockall A, Munari A, Avril N. New ways of assessing ovarian cancer response: metabolic imaging and beyond. Cancer Imaging. 2012;12(09):310–4.
16. Rockall AG, Avril N, Lam R, Iannone R, Mozley PD, Parkinson C, Bergstrom D, Sala E, Sarker SJ, Mcneish IA, Brenton JD. Repeatability of quantitative FDG-PET/CT and contrast-enhanced CT in recurrent ovarian carcinoma: test-retest measurements for tumor FDG uptake, diameter, and volume. Clin Cancer Res. 2014;20(10):2751–60.
17. Salem A, Salem AF, Al-Ibraheem A, Lataifeh I, Almousa A, Jaradat I. Evidence for the use PET for radiation therapy planning in patients with cervical cancer: a systematic review. Hematol Oncol Stem Cell Ther. 2011;4(4):173–81.

18. Schwarz JK, Lin LL, Siegel BA, Miller TR, Grigsby PW. 18-F-fluorodeoxyglucose-positron emission tomography evaluation of early metabolic response during radiation therapy for cervical cancer. Int J Radiat Oncol Biol Phys. 2008;72(5):1502–7.

19. Schwarz JK, Siegel BA, Dehdashti F, Grigsby PW. Association of posttherapy positron emission tomography with tumor response and survival in cervical carcinoma. JAMA. 2007;298(19):2289–95.

20. Scottish intercollegiate guidelines network. Management of cervical cancer. (SIGN guideline no 99). 2008. Available at: http://www.sign.ac.uk/guidelines/fulltext/99/index.html.

21. Scottish intercollegiate guidelines network. Management of epithelial ovarian cancer. (SIGN guideline no 135). 2013. Available at: http://www.sign.ac.uk/guidelines/fulltext/135/index.html.

22. Selman TJ, Mann C, Zamora J, Appleyard TL, Khan K. Diagnostic accuracy of tests for lymph node status in primary cervical cancer: a systematic review and meta-analysis. CMAJ. 2008;178(7):855–62.

23. Walentowicz-Sadlecka M, Malkowski B, Walentowicz P, Sadlecki P, Marszalek A, Pietrzak T, Grabiec M. The preoperative maximum standardized uptake value measured by 18F-FDG PET/CT as an independent prognostic factor of overall survival in endometrial cancer patients. Biomed Res Int. 2014;7:2014. doi:10.1155/2014/234813.

PET/CT in Gynaecological Malignancies: Pictorial Atlas

10

Sairah R. Khan and Tara Barwick

S.R. Khan
Department of Radiology, Imperial College Healthcare NHS Trust, Charing Cross Hospital, London, UK
e-mail: sairah.khan@imperial.nhs.uk

T. Barwick (✉)
Imperial College Healthcare NHS Trust, London, UK

Department of Surgery and Cancer, Imperial College, London, UK
e-mail: tara.barwick@imperial.nhs.uk

© Springer International Publishing Switzerland 2016
T. Barwick, A. Rockall (eds.), *PET/CT in Gynecological Cancers*,
Clinicians' Guides to Radionuclide Hybrid Imaging, DOI 10.1007/978-3-319-29249-6_10

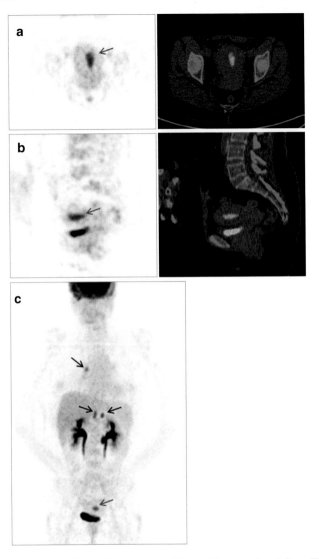

Fig. 10.1 Physiological endometrial activity: A 47-year-old was referred for a FDG PET/CT (PET and fused axial images (**a**), PET and fused sagittal images (**b**), MIP (**c**)) for staging of high-grade lymphoma which revealed intensely FDG-avid nodes both above and below the diaphragm (*black arrows*). Focal increased endometrial activity was noted on the MIP (**c**, *red arrow*) which in fact corresponded to linear increased activity on the axial and sagittal images (**a**, **b**, *red arrows*) in keeping with physiologic endometrial activity. The patient was menstruating at the time of the examination

Teaching Point Increased endometrial activity on the maximum intensity projection (MIP) must be carefully scrutinised on the multiplanar images and correlated with the patient's menstrual cycle. Linear increased endometrial activity during menstruation and ovulation is most in keeping with physiologic activity.

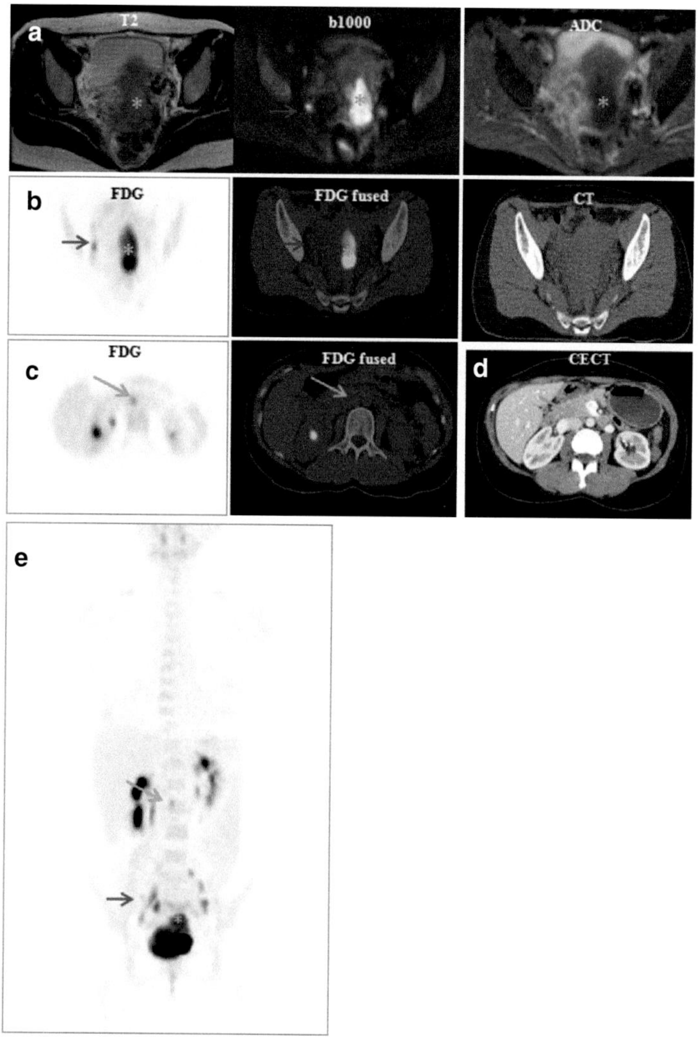

Fig. 10.2 Cervical cancer staging: A 39-year-old lady with FIGO stage IIIb cervical carcinoma. Pelvic MRI (**a**) demonstrates the primary tumour (*blue star*) and a small right-sided pelvic node (*red arrow*) not enlarged on the T2-weighted images but demonstrating restricted diffusion on diffusion weighted imaging (DWI). The primary tumour and right pelvic sidewall node were confirmed on FDG PET/CT (PET and fused axial images (**b**), MIP (**e**), *red arrows*), but also an aortocaval lymph node (PET and fused axial images (**c**), MIP (**e**), *green arrows*) which was occult on CECT (**d**) and outside the intended radiotherapy field. The PET changed the management to include aortic strip radiotherapy

Teaching Point FDG PET/CT is recommended in the routine staging of locally advanced cervical cancers >1B1 as it may identify disease beyond the pelvis.

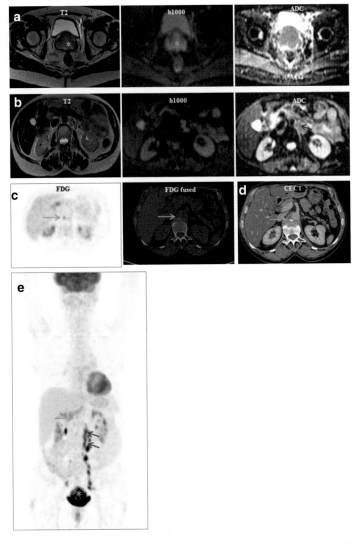

Fig. 10.3 Cervical cancer staging: A 56-year-old lady with a bulky cervical mass on pelvic MRI (**a**) (*blue star*) with bilateral parametrial, lower uterine segment and upper vaginal involvement in keeping with a FIGO stage IIb tumour. The MRI of the pelvis (**b**) also demonstrated bilateral external iliac and multiple retroperitoneal nodes (*red arrows*) extending up to the level of the renal hila on the left. FDG PET/CT (MIP (**e**)) confirmed the above sites of disease (*blue star & red arrows*), but in addition a metabolically active right retrocrural node (PET and fused axial images (**c**), MIP (**e**), *green arrows*) which was difficult to appreciate on the staging CECT (**d**) and outside the intended radiotherapy field. No metabolically active disease was demonstrated above the diaphragm

Teaching Point FDG PET/CT can help identify disease beyond the intended radiotherapy field and therefore change management. In addition, FDG PET/CT can be used for nodal IMRT contouring and radiotherapy planning.

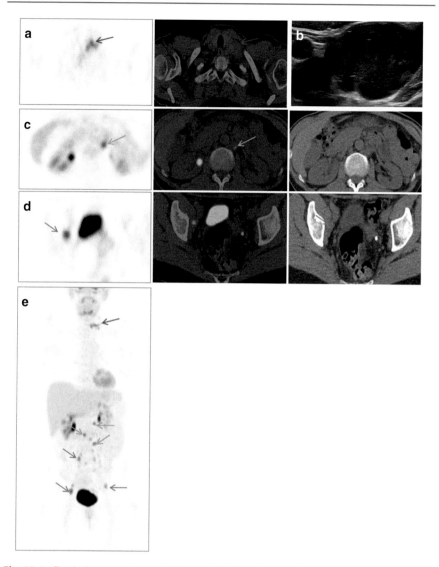

Fig. 10.4 Cervical cancer relapse: A 54-year-old lady with cervical carcinoma relapse thought to involve bilateral pelvic nodes only on conventional workup. The patient was being considered for salvage pelvic radiotherapy, but FDG PET/CT (PET and fused axial images (**a**), (**c**) and (**d**), MIP (**e**))demonstrated, in addition to the pelvic nodes (*blue arrows*), small retroperitoneal nodes (*green arrow*) and left supraclavicular nodes (*red arrow*). Ultrasound-guided biopsy of the left supraclavicular nodes (**b**) showed severely atypical epithelial cells of squamous cell origin in keeping with lymph node metastases

Teaching Point   FDG PET/CT can be helpful in cases of relapse thought to be suitable for salvage radiotherapy or exenterative surgery by identifying distant disease.

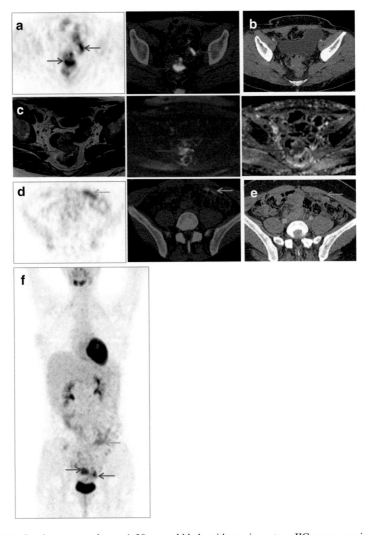

Fig. 10.5 Ovarian cancer relapse: A 30-year-old lady with previous stage IIC serous ovarian carcinoma, treated with total abdominal hysterectomy and bilateral salpingo-oopherectomy (TAH BSO) presented 18 months post surgery with increasing abdominal pain. FDG PET/CT (PET and fused axial images (**a**) and (**d**), MIP (**f**)) demonstrates focal increased metabolic activity within the sigmoid colon (*red arrows*) which corresponds to restricted diffusion on the MRI (**c**) in keeping with sigmoid serosal disease. In addition, FDG-avid peritoneal disease within the left iliac fossa (*green arrow*) was also noted. Both these sites of disease recurrence were difficult to appreciate on the CECT (**b**, **e**). The patient underwent salvage surgery with sigmoid colectomy for ovarian cancer recurrence

Teaching Point Focal increased activity within the bowel must be carefully scrutinised before being accounted as physiologic bowel activity which tends to be more diffuse. However, note peritoneal disease can mimic bowel activity on the PET, and the CT component of the PET needs to be reviewed carefully for small-volume peritoneal disease

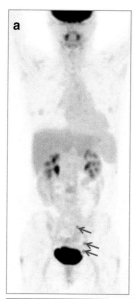

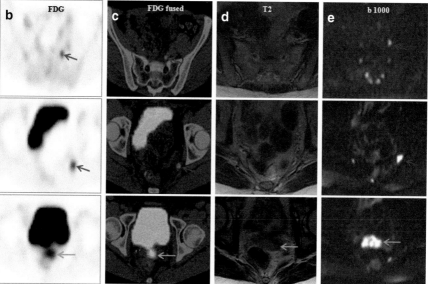

Fig. 10.6 Ovarian cancer relapse: A 35-year-old lady who previously underwent complete debulking for a high-grade serous ovarian carcinoma presented with a rising Ca-125. CECT did not show an obvious cause. The FDG PET/CT (MIP (**a**), PET and fused axial images column (**b**) and (**c**)) demonstrated three sites of subtle but definite pelvic nodal disease (*red arrows*) and a suspicious focus at the vaginal vault (*green arrow*). MRI of the pelvis confirmed these sites of disease on the *T2* (column **d**) and DWI (high **b** value column **e**)

Teaching Point   Closely scrutinise the vaginal vault for evidence of disease relapse as this is a site that can be masked by adjacent physiologic bladder activity.

Fig. 10.7 Endometrial cancer staging: A 60-year-old lady diagnosed with a carcinosarcoma of the uterus. The patient underwent a TAH BSO, and at the time of surgery, a suspicious node was sampled which proved to be a lymph node metastasis on histology: FIGO stage IIIC1. The postoperative staging FDG PET/CT (fused and PET axial images (**a–c**), MIP (**d**)) prior to pelvic radiotherapy demonstrated three further nodal sites of disease: left obturator (*blue arrow*), right common iliac (*red arrow*) and aortocaval nodes (*green arrow*). Prominent bowel activity secondary to metformin therapy was also noted. As a result of the FDG PET/CT, the patient was upstaged requiring para-aortic strip radiotherapy in addition to the original pelvic radiotherapy field

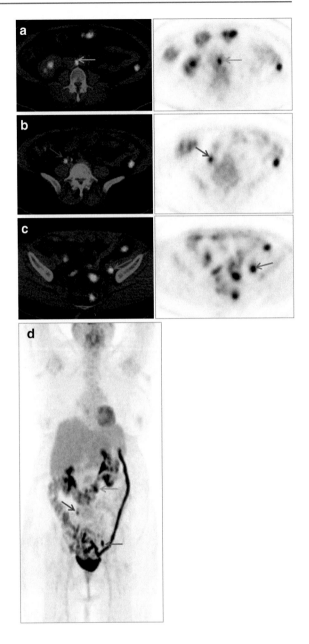

Teaching Point Although FDG PET/CT is not recommended in the routine staging of early stage endometrial cancer, in high-risk patients with known pelvic nodal disease, it can help delineate extra-pelvic disease.

Erratum to: Chapter 5, 6, 7 and 8 of PET/CT in Gynecological Cancers

Tara Barwick and Andrea Rockall

© Springer International Publishing Switzerland 2016
T. Barwick, A. Rockall (eds.), *PET/CT in Gynecological Cancers*,
Clinicians' Guides to Radionuclide Hybrid Imaging,
DOI 10.1007/978-3-319-29249-6

The below mentioned copyright comment has been included in Chapters 5, 6, 7 and 8:

Comment:

The content of this chapter has originally been published in: Szyszko: PET/CT in Esophageal and Gastric Cancer, © Springer 2016.

The updated original online version of the chapter can be found at

DOI 10.1007/978-3-319-29249-6_5
DOI 10.1007/978-3-319-29249-6_6
DOI 10.1007/978-3-319-29249-6_7
DOI 10.1007/978-3-319-29249-6_8

© Springer International Publishing Switzerland 2016
T. Barwick, A. Rockall (eds.), *PET/CT in Gynecological Cancers*,
Clinicians' Guides to Radionuclide Hybrid Imaging, DOI 10.1007/978-3-319-29249-6_11   E1

Index

© Springer International Publishing Switzerland 2016
T. Barwick, A. Rockall (eds.), *PET/CT in Gynecological Cancers*,
Clinicians' Guides to Radionuclide Hybrid Imaging, DOI 10.1007/978-3-319-29249-6